# Tendon Transfers in the Upper Limb

*Editor*

R. GLENN GASTON

# HAND CLINICS

www.hand.theclinics.com

*Consulting Editor*
KEVIN C. CHUNG

August 2016 • Volume 32 • Number 3

**ELSEVIER**

1600 John F. Kennedy Boulevard • Suite 1800 • Philadelphia, Pennsylvania, 19103-2899

http://www.theclinics.com

**HAND CLINICS Volume 32, Number 3**
**August 2016 ISSN 0749-0712, ISBN-13: 978-0-323-45967-9**

Editor: Jennifer Flynn-Briggs
Developmental Editor: Kristen Helm

*Hand Clinics* (ISSN 0749-0712) is published quarterly by Elsevier Inc., 360 Park Avenue South, New York, NY 10010-1710. Months of publication are February, May, August, and November. Business and Editorial Offices: 1600 John F. Kennedy Blvd., Ste. 1800, Philadelphia, PA 19103-2899. Customer Service Office: 3251 Riverport Lane, Maryland Heights, MO 63043. Periodicals postage paid at New York, NY and at additional mailing offices. Subscription price is $390.00 per year (domestic individuals), $687.00 per year (domestic institutions), $100.00 per year (domestic students/residents), $445.00 per year (Canadian individuals), $799.00 per year (Canadian institutions), $530.00 per year (international individuals), $799.00 per year (international institutions), and $256.00 per year (international and Canadian students/residents). Foreign air speed delivery is included in all *Clinics* subscription prices. All prices are subject to change without notice. **POSTMASTER:** Send address changes to *Hand Clinics*, Elsevier Health Sciences Division, Subscription Customer Service, 3251 Riverport Lane, Maryland Heights, MO 63043. Customer Service (orders, claims, online, change of address): Elsevier Health Sciences Division, Subscription **Customer Service, 3251 Riverport Lane, Maryland Heights, MO 63043. Tel: 1-800-654-2452 (U.S. and Canada); 314-447-8871 (outside U.S. and Canada). Fax: 314-447-8029. E-mail: journalscustomerservice-usa@elsevier.com (for print support); journalsonlinesupport-usa@elsevier.com (for online support).**

*Reprints.* For copies of 100 or more of articles in this publication, please contact the Commercial Reprints Department, Elsevier Inc., 360 Park Avenue South, New York, New York 10010-1710. Tel.: 212-633-3874; Fax: 212-633-3820; E-mail: reprints@elsevier.com.

*Hand Clinics* is covered in *MEDLINE/PubMed (Index Medicus), Current Contents/Clinical Medicine, EMBASE/Excerpta Medica,* and *ISI/BIOMED.*

# Contributors

## CONSULTING EDITOR

**KEVIN C. CHUNG, MD, MS**
Charles B.G. de Nancrede Professor of
Surgery, Professor of Plastic Surgery and
Orthopaedic Surgery, Chief of Hand
Surgery, University of Michigan Health
System, Assistant Dean for Faculty Affairs,
Associate Director of Global REACH,
University of Michigan Medical School,
Ann Arbor, Michigan

## EDITOR

**R. GLENN GASTON, MD**
Fellowship Director, OrthoCarolina Hand and
Upper Extremity Fellowship; Chief of Hand
Surgery, Carolinas Medical Center, Charlotte,
North Carolina

## AUTHORS

**ANCHAL BANSAL, BS**
Washington University School of Medicine,
St Louis, Missouri

**MICHAEL S. BEDNAR, MD**
Chief, Division of Hand Surgery; Professor,
Department of Orthopaedic Surgery and
Rehabilitation, Stritch School of Medicine,
Loyola University, Chicago, Illinois

**CHELSEA C. BOE, MD**
Resident Physician, Department of
Orthopedic Surgery, Mayo Clinic,
Rochester, Minnesota

**ROBERT CHRISTOPHER CHADDERDON, MD**
OrthoCarolina, Charlotte, North Carolina

**ANDRE EU-JIN CHEAH, MD, MBA**
Department of Orthopaedic Surgery, Robert A.
Chase Hand and Upper Limb Center, Stanford
University Medical Center, Redwood City,
California; Department of Hand and
Reconstructive Microsurgery, National
University Hospital, National University Health
System, Singapore, Singapore

**KEVIN C. CHUNG, MD, MS**
Charles B.G. de Nancrede Professor of
Surgery, Professor of Plastic Surgery and
Orthopaedic Surgery, Chief of Hand
Surgery, University of Michigan Health
System, Assistant Dean for Faculty Affairs,
Associate Director of Global REACH,
University of Michigan Medical School,
Ann Arbor, Michigan

**SHANE COOK, MD**
University of Iowa Hospitals and Clinics, Iowa City, Iowa

**RAFAEL J. DIAZ-GARCIA, MD**
Division of Plastic Surgery, Department of Surgery, Allegheny General Hospital, Allegheny Health Network; Clinical Assistant Professor of Plastic Surgery, University of Pittsburgh School of Medicine, Pittsburgh, Pennsylvania

**BASSEM T. ELHASSAN, MD**
Associate Professor of Orthopedics, College of Medicine, Mayo Clinic, Rochester, Minnesota

**JENNIFER ETCHESON, MS**
Department of Orthopaedic Surgery, Robert A. Chase Hand and Upper Limb Center, Stanford University Medical Center, Redwood City, California

**RYAN M. GARCIA, MD**
OrthoCarolina Hand Center, Charlotte, North Carolina

**R. GLENN GASTON, MD**
Fellowship Director, OrthoCarolina Hand and Upper Extremity Fellowship; Chief of Hand Surgery, Carolinas Medical Center, Charlotte, North Carolina

**CHARLES A. GOLDFARB, MD**
Professor and Vice Chairman, Department of Orthopaedic Surgery, St Louis Children's Hospital, Shriners Hospitals for Children, Washington University School of Medicine, St Louis, Missouri

**WARREN C. HAMMERT, MD**
Professor of Orthopaedic and Plastic Surgery; Chief, Division of Hand Surgery, Department of Orthopaedics and Rehabilitation, University of Rochester Medical Center, Rochester, New York

**DOUGLAS T. HUTCHINSON, MD**
Associate Professor, Department of Orthopaedics, University of Utah, Salt Lake City, Utah

**JONATHAN ISAACS, MD**
Herman M. and Vera H. Nachman Distinguished Research Professor; Professor and Chief, Division of Hand Surgery, Department of Orthopedic Surgery, Virginia Commonwealth University Health System, Richmond, Virginia

**DANIEL R. LEWIS, MD**
Clinical Instructor, OrthoCarolina Hand and Upper Extremity Fellowship, OrthoCarolina Hand Center; Orthopaedic Surgery Residency, Carolinas Medical Center, Charlotte, North Carolina

**ANDREW LIVERMORE, MD**
Orthopedic Surgery Resident, Department of Orthopedics and Rehabilitation, University of Wisconsin-Madison, Madison, Wisconsin

**BRYAN J. LOEFFLER, MD**
Clinical Instructor, OrthoCarolina Hand and Upper Extremity Fellowship, OrthoCarolina Hand Center; Orthopaedic Surgery Residency, Carolinas Medical Center, Charlotte, North Carolina

**GARY M. LOURIE, MD**
The Hand and Upper Extremity Center of Georgia, PC, Northside/Alpharetta Medical Campus, Alpharetta, Georgia

**CHRISTOPHER A. MAKAREWICH, MD**
Resident, Department of Orthopaedics, University of Utah, Salt Lake City, Utah

**MICHAEL BRODY O'SULLIVAN, MD**
Resident, Department of Orthopaedic Surgery, University of Connecticut Health Center, Farmington, Connecticut

**DAVID S. RUCH, MD**
Chief, Division of Hand Surgery, Department of Orthopedic Surgery, Duke University Medical Center, Durham, North Carolina

**HARDEEP SINGH, MD**
Resident, Department of Orthopaedic Surgery, University of Connecticut Health Center, Farmington, Connecticut

**JONATHAN L. TUETING, MD**
Chief, Hand and Upper Extremity Surgery; Associate Professor and Vice-Chair of Clinical Operations, University of Wisconsin School of Medicine and Public Health, Madison, Wisconsin

**OBINNA UGWU-OJU, MD**
Department of Orthopedic Surgery, Virginia Commonwealth University Health System, Richmond, Virginia

**LINDLEY B. WALL, MD**
Assistant Professor, Department of
Orthopaedic Surgery, St Louis Children's
Hospital, Shriners Hospitals for Children,
Washington University School of Medicine,
St Louis, Missouri

**DANIELLE WILBUR, MD**
Assistant Professor of Orthopaedic Surgery,
Department of Orthopaedics and
Rehabilitation, University of Rochester Medical
Center, Rochester, New York

**JENNIFER MORIATIS WOLF, MD**
Professor, Department of Orthopaedic
Surgery, University of Connecticut Health
Center, Farmington, Connecticut

**JEFFREY YAO, MD**
Department of Orthopaedic Surgery,
Robert A. Chase Hand and Upper Limb Center,
Stanford University Medical Center,
Redwood City, California

# Contents

Tendon transfers provide a substitute, either temporary or permanent, when function is lost due to neurologic injury in stroke, cerebral palsy or central nervous system lesions, peripheral nerve injuries, or injuries to the musculotendinous unit itself. This article reviews the basic principles of tendon transfer, which are important when planning surgery and essential for an optimal outcome. In addition, concepts for coapting the tendons during surgery and general principles to be followed during the rehabilitation process are discussed.

The transfer of tendons in the upper extremity is a powerful technique to restore function to a partially paralyzed hand. The biomechanical principles of muscle tension and tendon excursion dictate motor function both in the native as well as transferred states. Appropriately tensioning transferred tendons to maximize the function of the associated muscle remains an area of focused research. Newer methods of tendon coaptation have proven similar in strength to the standard Pulvertaft weave, affording more options to the surgeon.

Restoration of shoulder function in patients with brachial plexus injury can be challenging. Initial reported efforts were focused on stabilizing the shoulder, improving inferior subluxation and restoring abduction and flexion of the joint. Recent advancements and improved understanding of coordinated shoulder motion and the biomechanical properties of the muscles around the shoulder applicable to tendon transfer have expanded available surgical options to improve shoulder function, specifically external rotation. Despite the advances in reconstructive options, brachial plexus injury remains a serious problem that requires complex surgical solutions, prolonged recovery, and acceptance of functional loss.

Active elbow flexion is required to position the hand in space, and loss of this function is debilitating. Nerve transfers or nerve grafts to restore elbow flexion may be options when the target muscle is viable, but in delayed reconstruction when the biceps and brachialis are atrophied or damaged, muscle transfer options should be considered. Muscle transfer options are discussed with attention to the advantages and disadvantages of each transfer option.

> Radial nerve palsy typically occurs as a result of trauma or iatrogenic injury and leads to the loss of wrist extension, finger extension, thumb extension, and a reduction in grip strength. In the absence of nerve recovery, reconstruction of motor function involves tendon transfer surgery. The most common donor tendons include the pronator teres, wrist flexors, and finger flexors. The type of tendon transfer is classified based on the donor for the extensor digitorum communis. Good outcomes have been reported for most methods of radial nerve tendon transfers as is typical for positional tendon transfers not requiring significant power.

> The median nerve serves a crucial role in extrinsic and intrinsic motor and sensory function to the radial half of the hand. High median nerve injuries, defined as injuries proximal to the anterior interosseous nerve origin, therefore typically result in significant functional loss prompting aggressive surgical management. Even with appropriate recognition and contemporary nerve reconstruction, however, motor and sensory recovery may be inadequate. With isolated persistent high median nerve palsies, a variety of available tendon transfers can improve key motor functions and salvage acceptable use of the hand.

> Opposition is the placement of the thumb opposite the fingers into a position from which it can work. This motion requires thumb palmar abduction, flexion, and pronation, which are provided by the abductor pollicis brevis, flexor pollicis brevis (FPB), and opponens pollicis. In the setting of a median nerve palsy, this function is typically lost, although anatomic variations and the dual innervation of the FPB may prevent complete loss at times. There are multiple well described and accepted tendon transfers to restore opposition, none of which have been proven to be superior to the others.

> Ulnar nerve paralysis results in classic stigmata, including weakness of grasp and pinch, poorly coordinated flexion, and clawing of digits. Restoration of grasp is a key portion of the reconstructive efforts after loss of ulnar nerve function. Improving flexion at the metacarpophalangeal joint can be done by static and dynamic means, although only the latter can improve interphalangeal extension. Deformity and digital posture are more predictably corrected with surgical intervention. Loss of strength from intrinsic muscle paralysis cannot be fully restored with tendon transfer procedures. Preoperative patient education is paramount to success if realistic expectations are to be met.

> Power and tip pinch are an integral part of intrinsic hand function that can be significantly compromised with dysfunction of the ulnar nerve. Loss of power pinch is one

component that can significantly affect an individual's ability to perform simple daily tasks. Tip pinch is less affected, as this task has significant contributions from the median nerve. To restore power pinch, the primary focus must be on restoring the action of the adductor pollicis primarily, and if indicated the first dorsal interosseous muscle and flexor pollicis brevis.

Thumb hypoplasia is a component of radial longitudinal deficiency. The severity of hypoplasia can range from a slightly smaller thumb to a complete absence. Types II and IIIA hypoplastic thumbs are candidates for reconstruction to improve function, stability, and strength. There are 2 commonly used tendon transfers that can augment thumb opposition strength: the Huber abductor digiti minimi muscle transfer and the flexor digitorum superficialis opposition transfer. Both transfers use ulnar-sided structures to augment the thenar musculature. The Huber opposition transfer increases thenar bulk, but does not provide additional tissue for metacarpophalangeal stability.

The flexor carpi ulnaris to extensor carpi radialis brevis transfer and extensor pollicis longus rerouting combined with thenar release are 2 successful surgical interventions for children with spastic cerebral palsy. The goal of both procedures is to improve quality of life for patients who have previously failed conservative management, and the degree of expected improvement is predicated on several patient variables, making careful patient selection crucial for ensuring successful outcomes. Here, surgical technique is described; risk factors are discussed, and outcomes related to both procedures are presented.

# HAND CLINICS

**THE CLINICS ARE AVAILABLE ONLINE!**
Access your subscription at:
www.theclinics.com

# Preface

# An Update on Upper Extremity Tendon Transfers

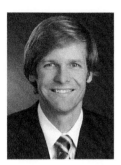

R. Glenn Gaston, MD
*Editor*

Tendon transfers have been a proven method of upper extremity reconstruction for well over 150 years. We are indebted to the pioneering hand surgeons such as Paul Brand, Richard Smith, Sterling Bunnell, Joseph Boyes, and many others who contributed the concepts that are still regarded as the guiding principles in tendon transfers performed today. While the anatomy, biomechanics, and fundamentals of tendon transfers haven't changed, many advances in tendon transfer surgery have been made over the last decade. In addition, our field is seeing tremendous growth in nerve repair, reconstruction, and nerve transfers, yet the need for tendon transfers to restore shoulder, elbow, wrist, and hand function will remain a necessary and powerful technique in regaining lost function of the arm.

In this issue of *Hand Clinics*, the core principles and biomechanics of upper extremity transfers are reviewed. Common transfers such as radial, median, and ulnar nerve tendon transfers are reviewed along with several pearls for success. Tendon transfers for specific conditions such as congenital hand deformity, rheumatoid arthritis,

and tetraplegia add completeness to the issue. Last, less well-described tendon transfers such as restoration of shoulder function and elbow flexion are discussed.

I am forever grateful to the outstanding contributions from such esteemed colleagues and friends who have made this issue not only possible but also so educational. You all sacrificed generous amounts of your time and energy and have created a wonderful work that I am confident many physicians will learn from for years to come: Thank You! I am most grateful, however, for the never-ending support of my wife, Krissa, and my three children, McLean, Myers, and Virginia, whose unwavering love and support will never go unappreciated.

R. Glenn Gaston, MD
OrthoCarolina
1915 Randolph Road
Charlotte, NC 28207, USA

E-mail address:
glenn.gaston@orthocarolina.com

# Principles of Tendon Transfer

Danielle Wilbur, MD[a], Warren C. Hammert, MD[b],*

## KEYWORDS

- Tendon transfer • Principles of tendon transfer • Restoration of nerve injury
- Reconstruction following nerve injury

## KEY POINTS

- Tendon transfers can be useful for restoration of function following peripheral nerve injuries or other conditions affecting the muscle/tendon units.
- Essential elements for successful tendon transfer include (A) supple joints: it is easier to prevent contractures than reverse them, so maintaining passive motion is preferable; (B) tissue equilibrium: timing of transfer is based on appropriate wound healing and scar maturation; (C) adequate strength and excursion; (D) one tendon for each function if possible; (E) straight line of pull; (F) expendable donor; (G) synergistic transfer (preferred, but not mandatory).
- If identified early, consider nerve reconstruction before embarking on tendon transfers.

## INTRODUCTION

Tendon transfers provide a substitute, either temporary or permanent, when function is lost due to peripheral nerve injuries or injuries to the musculotendinous unit itself or when function is imbalanced due to spasticity from neurologic injury in stroke, cerebral palsy, or central nervous system lesions. Understanding of the fundamental principles of tendon transfer allows the surgeon to establish, strengthen, or augment motor function that has been compromised. The tendon transfer itself is the release of a terminal or proximal tendon insertion from one functional muscle-tendon unit and reinsertion distally to restore lost or deficient muscle action.[1] In contrast, a tendon graft is transected both proximally and distally and used as an intercalary segment without preserving its neurovascular supply. A free muscle transfer involves transecting both the origin and the insertion of a musculotendinous unit and performing a distal revascularization and nerve repair

(see Garcia RM, Ruch DS: Free flap functional muscle transfers, in this issue). The first successful tendon transfers were performed in the foot to treat deformities caused during the polio endemic in Vienna in the 1880s by Carl Nicoladoni. This tendon transfer was expanded on by Codivilla, an Italian surgeon who performed a series of 30 tendon transfers and introduced the concept of muscle balance and need for preoperative assessment of donor muscle force.[1] The mid-1900s brought further advances by hand surgeons that bear the names of many transfers that are still performed today, including Mayer, Almquist, Steindler, Bunnel, Brand, Boyd, Omer, and Jones.[1–3]

It is essential to understand the fundamental elements that allow tendon transfer surgery to restore function. Only with understanding of the general principles of tendon transfer can the surgeon formulate an effective treatment algorithm specific to the patient's needs.

Disclosures: None.

[a] Department of Orthopaedics and Rehabilitation, University of Rochester Medical Center, 601 Elmwood Avenue, Box 665, Rochester, NY 14612, USA; [b] Division of Hand Surgery, Department of Orthopaedics and Rehabilitation, University of Rochester Medical Center, 601 Elmwood Avenue, Box 665, Rochester, NY 14612, USA
* Corresponding author.
*E-mail address:* Warren_Hammert@URMC.Rochester.edu

Hand Clin 32 (2016) 283–289
http://dx.doi.org/10.1016/j.hcl.2016.03.001
0749-0712/16/$ – see front matter © 2016 Elsevier Inc. All rights reserved.

## GENERAL PRINCIPLES OF TENDON TRANSFER
### Preoperative Assessment

Tendon transfers can be used to restore function to a joint, recover a specific motion across a joint, improve deformity, or to act as an internal splint to support partial function after distal nerve injury while awaiting recovery of a peripheral nerve injury.[4] Appropriate expectations of both the patient and the family must be ascertained before intervention with a careful assessment of the needs and goals of the patient and caretakers. A thorough evaluation of the patient is necessary to map out the functional deficits requiring transfer, establish which muscles are available for transfer, and determine the sensibility of the affected limb.[5] If the limb is insensate, the reduced sensory feedback will cause the brain to exclude these areas from functional activity and lead to suboptimal outcomes.[2] The time from injury, the type of injury, and success of previous treatment should be delineated. Electrodiagnostic studies may be helpful in determining the extent of motor loss of a limb and predicting further muscle recovery by the presence of polyphasics. Although clinical examination is sufficient in many instances, there are scenarios where electromyography (EMG) can greatly enhance the diagnostic capabilities. Evaluation of 2 muscles with similar function, such as pronator teres and pronator quadratus, can determine if one is expendable, such as with use of pronator teres transfer for wrist extension in radial nerve palsy. In addition, electrodiagnostic studies can clarify confounding pictures by demonstrating abnormal nerve patterns, such as Martin-Gruber connection or Riche-Cannieu connections, which may have implications on choice of transfer. Omer[4] described quantitative tests that should be performed during preoperative assessment, including voluntary muscle tests and measurements of range of motion, measurement of 2-point discrimination, gross grip and finger pinch strength tests, and timed pickup tests in cases involving median and/or ulnar nerve lesions. Realistic treatment goals must be agreed on by the patient, caretakers, surgeon, and rehabilitation team to ensure postoperative success. Unrealistic expectations that are not addressed before surgery can lead to frustration, lack of trust in the surgeon and rehabilitative team, and lack of perceived improvement in function.[6]

Tendon transfers are not time-sensitive, but when reconstruction for traumatic injuries is undertaken before motor end plate degeneration (typically 18 months from injury), nerve grafting or nerve transfers should be considered. If tendon transfers are performed early, end to side are preferable, because regeneration of the nerve will allow improvement in function. When performed late or when there is no chance of nerve recovery, either end-to-end or end-to-side transfers can be used at the surgeon's discretion.

### Tissue Equilibrium

The term tissue equilibrium was coined by Steindler and infers that maturation of the tissue bed has occurred before the timing of the tendon transfer.[3] The motion after a tendon transfer is hindered if there is an inadequate gliding surface due to scar tissue, residual edema, or residual joint stiffness. If the tissue bed is not pliable, the surgeon may consider flap coverage or developing a subcutaneous bed or tunnel through which to place the transfer in unscarred tissue. A silicone rod may also be used to create a smooth tunnel for later tendon transfer in a second-stage procedure. If these soft tissue constraints cannot be overcome, then another transfer should be chosen. Brand[7] described tunneling the tendon transfer with blunt dissection through natural subcutaneous tissue planes in order to find the path of least resistance for the tendon transfer. The use of curved incisions allows for the tendons to be placed under subcutaneous flaps and avoids placement of the rerouted tendons under the incision site.[7,8] Contraindications for an elective tendon transfer surgery include chronic wounds, contractures, or evidence of bony instability/nonunion below the area of the transfer.[4] The involved muscle will have diminished function in scar tissue because of the increased fibrotic tension and shorter residual fiber length of the muscle-tendon unit.[4]

### Mobile, Intercalary Joints

The basis upon which tendon transfers work is the application of an active motor unit across a passively mobile joint that has adequate stability. Dowd and Bluman[6] described the concept that tendon transfer procedures are most effective when they are used to correct supple deformities caused by dynamic muscular imbalances. The preoperative range of motion will never be exceeded by active motion following a tendon transfer; thus, maximal preoperative passive motion must be obtained. Preoperative rehabilitation with occupation and/or physical therapy is required to re-establish supple passive range of motion of the targeted joints.[1,9] Adjuvant therapies such as casting, stretching, dynamic orthotic use and/or surgical release of joint contractures before tendon transfer surgery may be necessary to achieve mobile joints.

On the contrary, hypermobile joints or excessive joint laxity can predispose tendon transfers to overcorrection. For example, patients undergoing tendon transfers into the lateral bands for intrinsic reconstruction may result in swan neck deformities in the presence of proximal interphalangeal joint hyperlaxity. Tendon transfers should be used with extreme caution in patients with known collagen disorders or hyperlaxity.

## Donor Muscle Properties

### Adequate strength

The donor tendon must have adequate strength to perform its intended function. Its strength must be at least a 4+ or 5 out of 5 on the Lovett scale (**Table 1**), because motor strength has been shown to lose one grade postoperatively.[1,10] An injured muscle with denervation that subsequently recovers is not an acceptable donor muscle due to the loss of strength that will result when it is transferred.[9]

When selecting a donor, the surgeon must take into consideration the work capacity of the muscles and choose one that is has sufficient strength to perform the recipient function. The work capacity of a muscle depends on both its fiber length and its cross-sectional area, given that work is a product of both force and distance. The work capacity of a given muscle is therefore proportional to its mass or volume. The relative tension capacities of the forearm and hand muscles were determined by dividing the tendon's fiber length (excursion) into the volume of each muscle to determine the cross-sectional area. The work capacities for hand and forearm muscles are seen in **Table 2**.[11]

Multiple factors contribute to the loss of muscle grade strength after tendon transfers, including the need for the muscle to pull through postoperative adhesions, differences in the line of pull between the donor and recipient muscle, and the tensioning of the donor muscle.[4,12] When muscles are tensioned during surgery, the surgeon attempts to mimic the natural resting length of the muscle. If the muscle is set at a length that is longer than the

| Table 2 Forearm muscle work capacity from strongest to weakest | |
| --- | --- |
| **Donor Muscle** | **m-kg** |
| FDS | 4.8 |
| FDP | 4.5 |
| FCU | 2 |
| BR | 1.9 |
| PT | 1.2 |
| FPL | 1.2 |
| FCR | 0.8 |
| PL | 0.1 |
| **Recipient Muscles** | **m-kg** |
| EDC | 1.7 |
| ECRL | 1.1 |
| ECU | 1.1 |
| ECRB | 0.9 |
| EIP | 0.5 |
| EPB | 0.1 |
| EPL | 0.1 |
| APL | 0.1 |

*Abbreviations:* APL, abductor pollicis longus; BR, brachioradialis; ECRB, extensor carpi radialis brevis; ECRL, extensor carpi radialis longus; ECU, extensor carpi ulnaris; EDC, extensor digitorum communis; EIP, extensor indicis propius; EPB, extensor pollicis brevis; EPL, extensor pollicis longus; FCR, flexor carpi radialis; FCU, flexor carpi ulnaris; FDP, flexor digitorum profundus; FDS, flexor digitorium superficialis; FPL, flexor pollicis longus; PL, palmaris longus; PT, pronator teres.

sarcomere's normal, natural resting length, then the muscle is placed on tension into the passive portion of a Blix curve, which corresponds to an inefficient biomechanical starting tension.[6] This corresponds to an inefficient starting tension biomechanically. Friden and Lieber[13,14] showed that when a donor muscle is overtensioned into the passive portion of the Blix curve, its potential contractile force decreases to 28% of its maximum force. This paradoxical loss of sarcomeres occurs when tension is too tight, resulting in a passive tenodesis effect of the transfer, causing a decrease in strength and function of the transfer.[12] This decrease in strength and function of the transfer is due to the inability to develop active tension in a stretched sarcomere, with a suboptimal interaction between myosin and actin filaments, producing suboptimal muscle force.[13] Thus, it is crucial to attempt to set the muscle length during tendon transfer at the resting length of the muscle, within its effective range of motion of the recipient joint that it is acting upon.[12]

It is also important to determine the amount of strength needed by the recipient muscle.

| Table 1 Lovett scale | |
| --- | --- |
| **Grade** | **Muscle Effort** |
| 0 | No movement |
| 1 | Contraction visible or palpable, fasciculations |
| 2 | Active movement with gravity eliminated |
| 3 | Active movement against gravity |
| 4 | Active muscle contraction against gravity with some resistance |
| 5 | Active muscle contraction against full resistance; full strength |

Transfers can broadly be grouped into either power or positional transfers. Power transfers would include transfers for restoring grasp, pinch, elbow flexion, and shoulder abduction/flexion and require more powerful donor muscles. Positional transfers, on the contrary, do not require such powerful muscle donors and include the restoration of thumb opposition and radial nerve function.

Last, the strength of the antagonist muscles needs to be considered to avoid overcorrection; this is especially true in cases of combined nerve palsy or global neurologic deficits where small alterations in forces can have profound impacts on the overall balance of the hand. The tensioning of the same tendon transfer will need to be dramatically different in a patient with cerebral palsy and substantial spasticity versus a patient with Charcot-Marie-Tooth and global neurologic weakness.

## Excursion

The tendon excursion, or amplitude, must be sufficient to restore the lost function of the recipient muscle and be similar to the tendon that it is replacing (**Table 3**). The amount of excursion that can be expected from tendons is directly related to its resting fiber length and can be estimated by the Boyes' 3,5,7 rule:

1. Wrist flexors and extensors: 33 mm
2. Finger extensors and extensor pollicis longus (EPL): 50 mm
3. Finger flexors: 70 mm

Augmentation of excursion can occur by the tenodesis effect in muscles that are in-phase or synergistic to each other. Wrist flexion and extension can add 20 to 30 mm of excursion (effective amplitude) through the tenodesis effect, facilitating finger extension and flexion, respectively.[2,15] Mobilization and release of the fascial attachments of the donor muscle as well as release of the donor muscle belly can also be used to increase the excursion of muscle, especially in the brachioradialis.[2,3,15] A muscle can also be converted from a monoarticular unit into a biarticular or multiarticular unit to benefit from the natural tenodesis effect to augment the amplitude of muscle excursion.[3]

### Expendable Donor

Boyes, and later Omer,[4] outlined the 50 different muscles that are used to activate movement in the hand and forearm and include (**Table 4**):

1. 5 muscles that control supination/pronation
2. 7 muscles that control movement of the hand at the wrist
3. 18 muscles that flex and extend the digits
4. 20 small muscles of the hand that contribute to precise motion

The redundancy in the number of muscles acting together to produce a motion allows one or more to

| Table 3<br>Tendon excursion | |
|---|---|
| Tendon | Excursion (mm) |
| Wrist flexors | 33 |
| Wrist extensors | 33 |
| Finger extensors | 50 |
| EPL | 50 |
| Finger flexors | 70 |

| Table 4<br>Muscles used to activate movement in the forearm/hand | |
|---|---|
| Action | Muscles |
| Supination/pronation | Pronator teres<br>Pronator quadratus<br>Supinator<br>Bicepsbrachii<br>Brachioradialis |
| Movement of hand at the wrist | FCU<br>FCR<br>Palmaris longus<br>ECRB<br>ECRL<br>ECU<br>EDC |
| Flexion/extension of digits | FDS × 4<br>FDP × 4<br>FDM<br>FPL<br>EDC × 4<br>EDQ<br>EIP<br>EPL<br>EPB<br>APL |
| Precise motion | Dorsal interossei × 4<br>Palmar interossei × 4<br>Lumbricals × 4<br>Thenar muscles<br>Hypothenar muscles<br>Adductor pollicis<br>Palmaris brevis |

*Abbreviations:* APL, abductor pollicis longus; ECRB, extensor carpi radialis brevis; ECRL, extensor carpi radialis longus; ECU, extensor carpi ulnaris; EDC, extensor digitorum communis; EDQ, extensor digiti quinti; EIP, extensor indicis proprius; EPB, extensor pollicis brevis; FDM, flexor digiti minimi; FDP, flexor digitorum profundus; FPL, flexor pollicis longus.

be used to augment function elsewhere. The donor tendon must be expendable, and its use must not result in considerable functional impairment after transfer, meaning the remaining muscles must have sufficient strength to account for the loss of function the donor used to provide. For example, there must be a sufficient wrist flexor remaining to flex the wrist after transfer for reconstruction of a radial nerve palsy.[3,4,9]

### One Tendon, One Function

When evaluating functional deficits and planning the muscles available for transfer, the surgeon must adhere to the one donor, one function rule. A single tendon cannot be expected to perform 2 functions, for example, to extend and flex the joint, without a subsequent loss of effectiveness because of the dissipation of the force and amplitude of the muscle by performing 2 opposite tasks.[2,3] In addition, it is difficult to use one tendon to perform 2 similar functions, such as extend the fingers and thumb. When 2 separate insertions are used, the tendon that is set with the greatest tension will be the active tendon and will overpower the other function.[1] One tendon may, however, be used to restore one function in multiple digits or multiple joints. For example, the flexor carpi radialis (FCR) or flexor carpi ulnaris (FCU) can be used to restore digital extension to all fingers simultaneously. Similarly, one tendon transfer may be used to influence more than one joint in the restoration of intrinsic function in ulnar nerve palsy by simultaneously improving metacarpophalangeal flexion and interphalangeal extension with the transfer of a donor through the lumbrical canal and into the lateral bands.

### Straight Line of Pull

The vector of motion of the tendon being transferred is crucial in creating functional motions across a joint and prevention of secondary deformities.[12] To maximize the force and efficiency of a transferred tendon, the line of pull from the donor motor site to the recipient insertion site should be as straight as possible without the use of redirectional pulleys whenever possible.[2,3]

### Synergism

The concept of synergy was advocated by Littler and relates to the concept that a transferred tendon's normal contractile period should be the same as the contractile period of the tendon that is being augmented. A synergistic transfer allows the muscle to contract during the expected motion, in a contraction sequence that is in phase with the recipient muscle.[1,6] Wrist flexion is synergistic with finger extension, and wrist extension is synergistic with finger flexion. Synergistic muscle contraction is easier for retraining muscle function after transfer, especially in children, who have greater cerebral plasticity than adults.[1,3] Use of preoperative dynamic EMG may help in determining appropriate muscles for transfer. Transfer of a wrist flexor for finger extension in radial nerve palsy is a common synergistic transfer. If this type of tendon transfer fails, the transfer can still function as a tenodesis effect if it is transferred in phase with the recipient muscle.[2]

### Surgical Technique

A variety of techniques have been described in the literature for coaptation of the donor and recipient tendons following tendon transfer. When choosing a coaptation style, the surgeon must determine whether an end-to-end type of attachment or an end-to-side type of coaptation can be used. This decision depends on multiple factors: length of tendon available for transfer, site of transfer, amount of soft tissue to cover the bulkiness of the tendon transfer, tensioning of the graft, and caliber of the tendons. The Pulvertaft weave can be used in both an end-to-side and a side-to-side transfer.[16] Pulvertaft tendon weave was originally described in his paper on flexor tendon fixation in the hand using the palmaris, plantaris, or extensor digitorum longus to the fourth toe as tendon grafts. He advocated the use of a fishmouth end-to-end interlacing stitch, first introduced by Bunnell, which is useful when the tendon and grafts have differing cross-sectional diameter. The remainder of the donor tendon is then interlaced through a series of 90° slits cut through the recipient tendon with cross stitches to interlock the tendons together.[16,17] The use of 4 to 5 weaves to increase the overall repair strength of the tendon weave, including in a Pulvertaft weave, was shown to be the strongest in peak load to failure and peak stress biomechanically in Gabuzda's study.[18] This biomechanical study also evaluated the tensile strength between 2 suturing techniques during an end-to-end tendon repair. A cross stitch was compared with horizontal mattress sutures, with cross-stitch patterns having a notable increase in pullout strength.[18]

The importance of high ultimate load to failure is crucial to allow early motion protocols to prevent tendon adhesion, limit postoperative complications, and potentiate improved clinical and functional outcomes.[19] Pulvertaft weaves usually fail at the knot site in the repair region due to the knot either slipping or pulling out through the tendon itself, whereas side-to-side techniques can fail via shearing through the fibers of the donor tendon, or via failure at the outer suture site.[19,20]

The tensile strength of the sutures used in a tendon weave and its effect on tendon vascularity have also been scrutinized. Tanaka and colleagues[21] introduced a new corner-stitch construct during the use of tendon weave fixation and compared this to the traditional central cross-suture design. This new design does not penetrate the full length of the tendon, and by avoiding full thickness stitches within the central substance of the tendon, theoretically poses less of a risk to the longitudinal intratendinous vasculature that is important for the revascularization of tendon grafts without sacrificing tensile strength. Despite the theories behind preservation of intratendinous blood supply by peripheral placement of sutures, Gelberman and colleagues[22,23] showed no effect on the vascularity of the proximal tendon in a tendon graft with horizontal mattress suture repair.

Side-to-side tendon repairs have been advocated in children because of the smaller caliber of tendons.[20] Alternative coaptation methods in addition to side-to-side and Pulvertaft weaves include the lasso and the loop-tendon suture technique.[16,20] The lasso technique of Bidic and colleagues[20] is useful for tendon transfers proximal to the carpal tunnel in the volar forearm and proximal to zone 5 on the dorsal hand/forearm. It has a maximal load to failure similar to that of the Pulvertaft weave, is stronger than the side-to-side technique, and requires less tendon length and half the weave time of the Pulvertaft weave.[20] The loop-tendon suture technique described by Kim and colleagues[16] had a higher ultimate tensile load than end-weave suture techniques and is beneficial in its ease of technique, ease of revision when readjusting tension due to removal of only one loop of tendon, ability to set independent tension of the finger cascade, as required in an FCR to EDC tendon transfer, and the lack of damage to the donor or recipient tendon due to lack of longitudinal slit incisions for weaving. Disadvantages to all tendon transfer coaptation methods include bulkiness of the tendon graft site that may increase friction and smooth gliding of tendons and its ability to be used in places other than the dorsal hand or within the forearm.[16]

### Rehabilitation

In general, rehabilitation following tendon transfers involves a period of immobilization followed by therapy to learn how to use the transfer. Synergistic transfers are easier to learn and are the authors' preference when possible. There may be some benefit to having the patient see the therapists before surgery to begin learning what will be involved with the postoperative therapy, such as learning to focus on a specific muscle motion that will be used in the transfer (isolating flexion of flexor digitorum superficialis [FDS] to learn how to activate for finger extension after transfer). The more complicated the transfer, the more time and effort to learn to use the transfer. In addition, the rehabilitation process may vary between static and dynamic transfers for specific conditions, such as correction of clawing associated with ulnar nerve palsy.

## REFERENCES

1. Fitoussi F, Bachy M. Tendon lengthening and transfer. Orthop Traumatol Surg Res 2015;101(1): S149–57.
2. Solomons M. Disorders of the hand: tendon transfers. In: Trail IA, Fleming AN, editors. Disorders of the hand volume 2: hand reconstruction and nerve compression. London: Springer; 2015. p. 33–55.
3. Ingari JV, Green DP. Green's operative hand surgery. In: Wolfe SW, Hotchkiss RN, Pederson WC, et al, editors. Green's operative hand surgery. 6th edition. Philadelphia: Elsevier Inc; 2011. p. 1075–92.
4. Omer GE. Tendon transfers for traumatic nerve injuries. J Am Soc Surg Hand 2004;4(3):214–26.
5. Ratner JA, Peljovich A, Kozin SH. Update on tendon transfers for peripheral nerve injuries. J Hand Surg Am 2010;35A(8):1371–81.
6. Dowd T, Bluman EM. Tendon transfers—how do they work? Planning and implementation. Foot Ankle Clin N Am 2014;19:17–27.
7. Brand P. Biomechanics of tendon transfer. Orthop Clin North Am 1974;5:205–30.
8. Omer G. The technique and timing of tendon transfers. Orthop Clin North Am 1974;5:243–52.
9. Kozin SH. Tendon transfers for radial and median nerve palsies. J Hand Ther 2005;18:208–15.
10. Omer GJ. Evaluation and reconstruction of the forearm and hand after traumatic peripheral nerve injuries. J Bone Joint Surg Am 1968;50A: 1454–78.
11. Brand P, Beach R, Thompson D. Relative tension and potential excursion of muscles in the forearm and hand. J Hand Surg Am 1981;6A:209–19.
12. Peljovich A, Ratner JA, Marino J. Update of the physiology and biomechanics of tendon transfer surgery. J Hand Surg Am 2010;35A(8):1365–9.
13. Lieber RL, Murray WM, Clark DL, et al. Biomechanical properties of the brachioradialis muscle: implications for surgical tendon transfer. J Hand Surg Am 2005;30A(2):273–82.
14. Friden J, Lieber RL. Evidence for muscle attachment at relatively long lengths in tendon transfer surgery. J Hand Surg Am 1998;23A:105–10.

15. Seiler JG, Desai MJ, Payne SH. Tendon transfers for radial, median, and ulnar nerve palsy. J Am Acad Orthop Surg 2013;21(11):675–84.

16. Kim SH, Chung MS, Baek GH, et al. A loop-tendon suture for tendon transfer or graft surgery. J Hand Surg Am 2007;32A(3):367–72.

17. Pulvertaft R. Tendon grafts for flexor tendon injuries in the fingers and thumb: a study of technique and results. J Bone Joint Surg Am 1956;38B:175–94.

18. Gabuzda G, Lovallo JL, Nowak MD. Tensile strength of the end-weave flexor tendon repair. J Hand Surg Am 1994;19B(3):397–400.

19. Brown SHM, Hentzen ER, Kwan A, et al. Mechanical strength of the side-to-side versus Pulvertaft weave tendon repair. J Hand Surg Am 2010;35A(4):540–5.

20. Bidic SM, Varshney A, Ruff MD, et al. Biomechanical comparison of lasso, Pulvertaft weave, and side-by-side tendon repairs. Plast Reconstr Surg 2009; 124(2):567–71.

21. Tanaka T, Zhao C, Ettema AM, et al. Tensile strength of a new suture for fixation of tendon grafts when using a weave technique. J Hand Surg Am 2006; 31A(6):982–6.

22. Gelberman R, Khabie V, Cahill C. The revascularization of healing flexor tendons in the digital sheath. A vascular injection study in dogs. J Bone Joint Surg Am 1991;73A:868–81.

23. Gelberman R, Chu C, Williams C, et al. Angiogenesis in healing autogenous flexor tendon grafts. J Bone Joint Surg Am 1992;74A:1207–16.

# Biomechanics of Tendon Transfers

Andrew Livermore, MD[a], Jonathan L. Tueting, MD[b],*

## KEYWORDS

- Biomechanics • Tendon transfer • Sarcomere • Excursion • Tendon coaptation

## KEY POINTS

- Tendon transfers depend on the tension and excursion capabilities of the transferred muscle.
- Anatomic charts have been created allowing comparison of potential donor-recipient muscle pairs.
- Tensioning the transferred muscle determines its functional capacity for force generation. Although work is being done to quantitate this, it remains poorly understood.
- A single transferred muscle controlling multiple tendons, either in parallel or series, presents unique challenges to the surgeon and patient.
- Multiple coaptation methods have been shown to be similar to the standard Pulvertaft weave.

## INTRODUCTION

This article explores the biomechanical principles governing tendon transfers in the upper extremity. The intricate mechanics of the hand are often taken for granted in health, but even slight aberrations can greatly impair function. In the devastating setting of a partially paralyzed hand, a firm understanding of these mechanics can allow the surgeon to redirect forces from uninjured areas to restore function of the hand. Although many of the mechanical principles remain as first described by the founders of tendon transfer, such as Bunnell and Boyes, vast improvements in the understanding of anatomic and biochemical properties of upper extremity muscles by the likes of Brand and Lieber have pushed the field to exciting new places and uncovered new areas for research.

## BIOMECHANICS FUNDAMENTALS
### Balance and Synergy

When function has been compromised in a hand due to acquired or congenital neuromuscular deficits, various surgical options may exist for functional restoration, including early reestablishment of nerve function (nerve transfer or reconstruction) or subsequent substitution for muscle weakness via tendon transfer. The former is beyond the scope of this article and is not addressed here. In the absence of reversing paralysis, the hand surgeon is tasked with redistributing the remaining strength in the limb.

Achieving balance is the ultimate goal of tendon transfer surgery. Balance does not imply equal strength on either side of a joint, but rather sufficient strength to ensure stability. For example, in restoring wrist extension following a radial nerve palsy, the extension moment created must be adequate to balance the flexion moment created by the finger flexors. This creates a stable wrist joint, maximizing the hand's ability for more distal activity.

The concept of synergism is integrally related to balance. It denotes 2 or more muscle functions that amplify the effect of the others, whether simultaneously or sequentially. Active synergism involves 2 concurrent actions. A natural pairing in the upper extremity is that of wrist extension with finger flexion,

Disclosures: The authors have nothing to disclose.
[a] Department of Orthopedics and Rehabilitation, University of Wisconsin-Madison, 1685 Highland Avenue, Madison, WI 53705, USA; [b] Hand and Upper Extremity Surgery, University of Wisconsin School of Medicine and Public Health, UWMF Centennial Building, 6th Floor, 1685 Highland Avenue, Madison, WI 53705, USA
* Corresponding author.
E-mail address: tueting@ortho.wisc.edu

Hand Clin 32 (2016) 291–302
http://dx.doi.org/10.1016/j.hcl.2016.03.011

as well as wrist flexion and finger extension. Maintaining synergistic relationships during tendon transfer, such as wrist flexors to finger extensors for radial nerve palsy, facilitates retraining in the postoperative period, as these muscle groups are typically fired together. This is especially relevant in older patients, and less so in children, whose neuroplasticity allows rapid adaptation to new muscle function.[1]

Sequential synergism relates to the passive stretch placed into a muscle by the active contraction of a complementary muscle. This storing of potential energy in a muscle places it in a more mechanically advantageous position to effect strong contraction and is essential in efficient function of skeletal muscle (**Fig. 1**). We explore this further in the next section.

## Muscle Mechanics

Fundamental to understanding tendon transfers is an understanding of the mechanics of the native musculotendinous unit. Brand[2] pointed out that each muscle can be described by just 2 parameters, its potential for generating tension, and its excursion, or the distance and direction over which this tension is exerted.

### Tension

Tension in skeletal muscle comes from 2 primary sources. Most commonly considered is active contraction, though equally important is passive elastic recoil of a stretched muscle. The functional unit of active contraction is the sarcomere, which is under voluntary nervous control (**Fig. 2**). It is composed of filaments of actin emanating from adjacent Z plates and interweaving with the intervening myosin filaments. When activated, the myosin filaments pull the actin filaments and subsequently the attached Z plates closer together, causing contraction and, therefore, tension. Sarcomeres are arranged in series to form fibers on a macroscopic level, and the

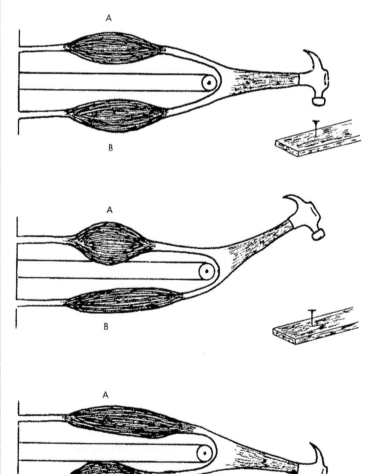

**Fig. 1.** When the hammer strikes, it is using both the active contraction of B plus the elastic recoil in B that has been put into it by A. (*From* Brand PW, Hollister A. Clinical mechanics of the hand. Second edition. St Louis (MO): Mosby Year Book; 1993. p. 19; with permission.)

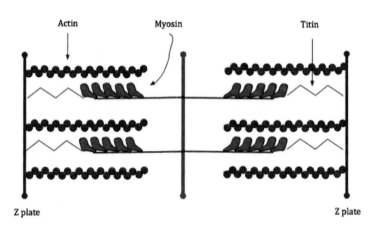

Actin          Myosin          Titin

Z plate                              Z plate

Fig. 2. The sarcomere. When stimulated by a nerve impulse, myosin pulls actin filaments and their attached Z plates closer together, causing muscle contraction. Titin is passively stretched when the sarcomere is lengthened.

observed contractile behavior of muscle fibers is a direct result of sarcomere contraction on an individual level. Prior studies have shown that a sarcomere length of 2.6 to 2.8 µm in human muscle is optimal for force generation.[3] Further, it has long been known that muscle cross-sectional area directly relates to a muscle's ability to generate tension, with a figure of approximately 3.6 kg/cm$^2$.[4]

Of fundamental importance to tendon transfer is the relationship of sarcomere length to contraction potential. At resting length (the length of a sarcomere in a muscle at rest, while the parent muscle is neither on stretch nor contracted), the potential for force generation is greatest (**Fig. 3**, center). This is due to the maximal overlap of myosin and actin and occurs at a length midway along the range from fully stretched to fully contracted. As

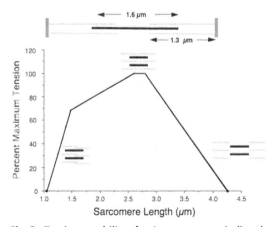

Fig. 3. Tension capability of a given sarcomere is directly related to its length, as this is the primary determinant of the degree of actin and myosin overlap. (*From* Friden J, Lieber RL. Mechanical considerations in the design of surgical reconstructive procedures. J Biomech 2002;35(8):1039–45; with permission.)

the sarcomere is stretched beyond its resting length, the overlap of myosin on actin is decreased and thus fewer bonds are available to generate contraction, and tension decreases (see **Fig. 3**, right). When shortened beyond resting length, maximal overlap is still in effect, but the sarcomere cannot shorten further, again limiting its tension capability (see **Fig. 3**, left). This relationship of length to tension is essential for successful tendon transfer, as is detailed shortly.

Muscles also have inherent elastic tendencies, independent of voluntary control. Elasticity of muscle causes it to inherently shorten when stretched or released from tension in the case of rupture. This property is due both to connective tissue external to the muscle, and more importantly to an intrasarcomeric cytoskeletal protein known as titin.[5] Elastic behaviors have a complex interplay with active contraction as it relates to tension generation. First, as a muscle is stretched, elastic recoil prevents overstretch of the sarcomere, maintaining it within a functional range of length. Second, as a muscle contracts, increasing elastic tension builds up in the antagonist muscle, resisting further contraction.

This interplay can be diagrammed with the well-known Blix curve, as first described by Magnus Blix in the late 1800s.[1] It consists of 2 additive length-tension curves for an individual muscle. The first curve is active contraction versus length, whereas the second is elastic recoil versus length, and their summated curve generally represents the tension in a muscle as it contracts from a lengthened position (**Fig. 4**A). Brand[1] went on to consider the curve in the setting of an antagonist muscle that is passively stretched during contraction of the muscle in question (**Fig. 4**B). Essentially, the elastic curve of the antagonist is subtracted from the active contraction of the primary muscle. This generates a composite curve of a muscle in

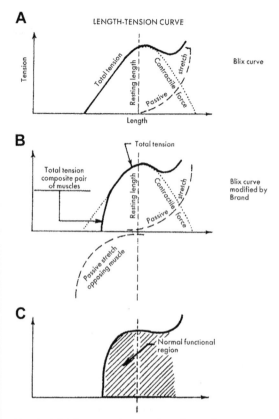

**Fig. 4.** (*A*) Blix curve, integrating the active contraction and elastic recoil. (*B*) Brand curve integrating the above with the elastic curve of the opposing muscle subtracted from the output of the primary muscle. (*C*) Final approximate shape of the curve in site in intact limb. (*From* Brand PW, Hollister A. Clinical mechanics of the hand. Second edition. St Louis (MO): Mosby Year Book; 1993. p. 20; with permission.)

situ (**Fig. 4**C). This interaction produces a shorter range of contraction than the muscle in isolation, but also augments the tension output of the measured muscle.

### Excursion

The capability of a muscle to do work is determined not only by its ability to generate tension, but the distance over which that tension can be exerted. This is known as excursion. This value varies from muscle to muscle in its native state, but the following distances have been generally accepted as being functional[6]:

Wrist extensors and flexors: 33 mm.
Finger extensors and extensor pollicis longus (EPL): 50 mm.
Finger flexors: 70 mm.

Wrist flexion and extension can add another 20 to 30 mm to the latter 2 motions via the

tenodesis effect. This explains why it not unreasonable to expect a tendon with a 25-mm excursion to fully substitute for finger extension.

Excursion is generally an inherent property of a given muscle based on the length and orientation of that muscle's fibers. With certain muscles, excursion can be improved by the surgeon via soft tissue releases, although the relationship may not be as direct as previously considered.[7] Considering the excursion of a transferred tendon is vital in planning a transfer.

### Planning

Planning is essential to achieve a successful outcome for an individual patient. First, a careful log of functional deficits must be created by detailed strength examination and closely observing the patient using his or her hand. It is important to include the patient in this conversation and take into account the deficits that are most devastating to the patient's life and vocation. Once the deficits are first listed and then prioritized in this way, the surgeon can consider which available muscles will best be suited to restore function in terms of tension capacity and excursion.

Modern hand surgeons owe much to the pioneering anatomic cataloging performed by Brand (**Table 1**).[4] He classified all the muscles below the elbow according to their fiber length, which corresponds to excursion, and cross-sectional area (reformulated as tension fraction), a surrogate for tension capacity. This was the first anatomic catalog of the 2 most important parameters for tendon transfer and gave surgeons more objective data from which to make their selection. Lieber and colleagues[8] took this anatomic study 1 step further. They also performed an intricate architectural study of the forearm and hand musculature and developed a difference index, which is a numerical value calculated for each muscle in relation to all the others in the forearm that quantifies the architectural (fiber length and cross section) similarity between 2 muscles (**Table 2**). This table provides surgeons with more objective data on how a given donor muscle relates to the paralyzed recipient.

### MUSCLE CHANGES FOLLOWING TRANSFER

Conventional wisdom states that a transferred muscle will lose one grade of strength (ie, from 5/5–4/5) following transfer. This is an oversimplification but does underscore the fact that a transferred muscle will likely not, for a number of reasons, develop the full working capacity of the muscle it is replacing. This may be due to reduced muscle tension or decreased excursion.

**Table 1**
**Anatomic catalog of forearm musculature**

| Mean Resting Fiber Length, cm | | Mass Fraction, % | | Tension Fraction, % | |
|---|---|---|---|---|---|
| BR | 16.1 | BR | 7.7 | Supinator | 7.1 |
| ECRL | 9.3 | ECRL | 6.5 | FCU | 6.7 |
| FDS (ring finger) | 7.3 | FCU | 5.6 | PT | 5.5 |
| FDS (index finger) | 7.2 | PT | 5.6 | ECU | 4.5 |
| FDS (little finger) | 7.0 | ECRB | 5.1 | ECRB | 4.2 |
| FDS (middle finger) | 7.0 | FDS (middle finger) | 4.7 | FCR | 4.1 |
| FDP (ring finger) | 6.8 | FDP (middle finger) | 4.4 | ECRL | 3.5 |
| FDP (index finger) | 6.6 | FCR | 4.2 | FDP (middle finger) | 3.4 |
| FDP (middle finger) | 6.6 | FDP (ring finger) | 4.1 | FDS (middle finger) | 3.4 |
| Lumbrical (middle finger) | 6.6 | ECU | 4.0 | First DI | 3.2 |
| FDP (little finger) | 6.2 | Supinator | 3.8 | APL | 3.1 |
| ECRB | 6.1 | FDP (index finger) | 3.5 | AP | 3.0 |
| EDC (middle finger) | 6.0 | FDP (little finger) | 3.4 | FDP (ring finger) | 3.0 |
| Lumbrical (ring finger) | 6.0 | FPL | 3.2 | PQ | 3.0 |
| EDC (little finger) | 5.9 | FDS (ring finger) | 3.0 | FDP (little finger) | 2.8 |
| EDQ | 5.9 | FDS (index finger) | 2.9 | FDP (index finger) | 2.7 |
| FPL | 5.9 | APL | 2.8 | FPL | 2.7 |
| EDC (ring finger) | 5.8 | EDC (middle finger) | 2.2 | Second DI | 2.5 |
| EPL | 5.7 | AP | 2.1 | BR | 2.4 |
| EDC (index finger) | 5.5 | EDC (ring finger) | 2.0 | Third DI | 2.0 |
| EIP | 5.5 | PQ | 1.8 | FDS (index finger) | 2.0 |
| Lumbrical (index finger) | 5.5 | EPL | 1.5 | FDS (ring finger) | 2.0 |
| FCR | 5.2 | First DI | 1.4 | ODQ | 2.0 |
| PT | 5.1 | FDS (little finger) | 1.3 | EDC (middle finger) | 1.9 |
| PL | 5.0 | EDQ | 1.2 | OP | 1.9 |
| Lumbrical (little finger) | 4.9 | PL | 1.2 | Fourth DI | 1.7 |
| APL | 4.6 | ADQ | 1.1 | EDC (ring finger) | 1.7 |
| ECU | 4.5 | EDC (index finger) | 1.1 | ADQ | 1.4 |
| EPB | 4.3 | EIP | 1.1 | EPL | 1.3 |
| FCU | 4.2 | EDC (little finger) | 1.0 | FPB | 1.3 |
| ADQ | 4.0 | OP | 0.9 | First PI | 1.3 |

(continued on next page)

**Table 1**
*(continued)*

| Mean Resting Fiber Length, cm | | Mass Fraction, % | | Tension Fraction, % | |
|---|---|---|---|---|---|
| APB | 3.7 | FPB | 0.9 | Second PI | 1.2 |
| AP | 3.6 | APB | 0.9 | PL | 1.2 |
| FPB | 3.6 | Second DI | 0.7 | APB | 1.1 |
| FDQ | 3.4 | EPB | 0.7 | EDC (index finger) | 1.0 |
| PQ | 3.0 | Third DI | 0.6 | EDQ | 1.0 |
| Supinator | 2.7 | ODQ | 0.6 | EIP | 1.0 |
| First DI | 2.5 | Fourth DI | 0.5 | Third PI | 1.0 |
| OP | 2.4 | First PI | 0.4 | EDC (little finger) | 0.9 |
| Second PI | 1.7 | Second PI | 0.4 | FDS (little finger) | 0.9 |
| Third DI | 1.5 | FDQ | 0.3 | EPB | 0.8 |
| Fourth DI | 1.5 | Third PI | 0.3 | FDQ | 0.4 |
| ODQ | 1.5 | Lumbrical (index finger) | 0.2 | Lumbrical (index finger) | 0.2 |
| First PI | 1.5 | Lumbrical (middle finger) | 0.2 | Lumbrical (middle finger) | 0.2 |
| Third PI | 1.5 | Lumbrical (ring finger) | 0.1 | Lumbrical (ring finger) | 0.1 |
| Second DI | 1.4 | Lumbrical (little finger) | 0.1 | Lumbrical (little finger) | 0.1 |

Surrogates for excursion (fiber length) and tension (tension fraction) are described for each muscle. The "mass fraction" of a muscle = the mass of the fleshy part of the muscle divided by the total mass of all the muscles below the elbow × 100. The "tension fraction" is the cross-sectional area of all the fibers of a muscle divided by the sum of the cross-sectional areas of all the muscle fibers below the elbow × 100.

*Abbreviations:* ADQ, abductor digiti quinti; AP, adductor pollicis; APB, abductor pollicis brevis; APL, abductor pollicis longus; BR, brachioradialis; DI, dorsal interosseous; ECRB, extensor carpi radialis brevis; ECRL, extensor carpi radialis longus; EDC, extensor digitorum communis; EDQ, extensor digiti quinti; ECU, extensor carpi ulnaris; EIP, extensor indicis proprius; EPB, extensor pollicis brevis; EPL, extensor pollicis longus; FCR, flexor carpi radialis; FCU, flexor carpi ulnaris; FDP, flexor digitorum profundus; FDQ, flexor digit quinti; FDS, flexor digitorum superficialis; FPB, flexor pollicis brevis; FPL, flexor pollicis longus; ODQ, opponens digiti quinti; OP, opponens pollicis; PI, palmar interosseous; PL, palmaris longus; PQ, pronator quadratus; PT, pronator teres.

*From* Brand PW, Beach MA, Thompson DE. Relative tension and potential excursion of muscles in the forearm and hand. J Hand Surg Am 1981;6(3):209–19; with permission.

## Tension Capacity

Because muscle tension is a function of cross-sectional area, simply transferring a tendon should not change the inherent tension capacity of a muscle, assuming the blood and nervous supply remain intact. This assumes appropriate tensioning of the muscle-tendon unit, which as is shown shortly, cannot be easily assumed. Nevertheless, the functional demand placed on a transferred muscle may be higher than what was previously expected from the muscle, resulting in relative weakness. Muscles can be strengthened following transfer, however, and this can be greatly facilitated by postoperative therapy.[1] However, it remains essential to wisely select well-matched muscles for transfer, as no amount of therapy can overcome a muscle that is inherently much weaker than the muscle it is being asked to replace.

## Excursion

Limits to excursion are likely a more important cause of weakness after tendon transfer than a change in muscle tension. This is partially related to the mismatch of excursion of the native muscle to the vector and excursion of the substitute. As with tension, this disparity can be mitigated by thoughtful selection of a donor muscle that is reasonably matched in terms of line of pull and overall excursion.

Another important postoperative limit to excursion is that of resistance. Native tendons glide smoothly in synovial sheaths in the case of flexor tendons, or in beds of loose areolar tissue rich in lubricating mucopolysaccharides in the case of nonsynovial tendons.[2] Scar, whether from an injury or surgery, can be devastating if not respected and appropriately accounted for. As was previously outlined, Boyes[6] has advocated waiting for "tissue equilibrium" before performing a transfer, so as to limit devastating adhesions. This includes allowing fractures to heal, swelling to resolve, scars to soften, and any necessary skin grafting to mature.[9]

It is necessary to consider the tissue bed in which the transferred tendon will lie. Ideally, it will rest in the subcutaneous tissue above the deep fascia. Scarring to this fatty tissue will be minimal

**Table 2**
**Difference index of forearm muscles**

| | FCR | FCU | PL | ECRB | ECRL | ECU | FDSI | FDSM | FDSR | FDSS | FDPI | FDPM | FDPR | FDPS | FPL | EDCI | EDCM | EDCR | EDCS | EDQ | EIP | EPL | PT | PQ | BR | FDS | FDP | EDC |
|---|---|---|---|---|---|---|---|---|---|---|---|---|---|---|---|---|---|---|---|---|---|---|---|---|---|---|---|---|
| FCR | 0.00 | — | — | — | — | — | — | — | — | — | — | — | — | — | — | — | — | — | — | — | — | — | — | — | — | — | — | — |
| FCU | 0.63 | 0.00 | — | — | — | — | — | — | — | — | — | — | — | — | — | — | — | — | — | — | — | — | — | — | — | — | — | — |
| PL | 0.63 | 1.23 | 0.00 | — | — | — | — | — | — | — | — | — | — | — | — | — | — | — | — | — | — | — | — | — | — | — | — | — |
| ECRB | 0.36 | 0.65 | 0.87 | 0.00 | — | — | — | — | — | — | — | — | — | — | — | — | — | — | — | — | — | — | — | — | — | — | — | — |
| ECRL | 0.94 | 1.40 | 0.94 | 0.86 | 0.00 | — | — | — | — | — | — | — | — | — | — | — | — | — | — | — | — | — | — | — | — | — | — | — |
| ECU | 0.27 | 0.39 | 0.90 | 0.33 | 1.06 | 0.00 | — | — | — | — | — | — | — | — | — | — | — | — | — | — | — | — | — | — | — | — | — | — |
| FDSI | 0.31 | 0.62 | 0.78 | 0.56 | 0.99 | 0.34 | 0.00 | — | — | — | — | — | — | — | — | — | — | — | — | — | — | — | — | — | — | — | — | — |
| FDSM | 0.42 | 0.46 | 1.02 | 0.38 | 1.00 | 0.23 | 0.37 | 0.00 | — | — | — | — | — | — | — | — | — | — | — | — | — | — | — | — | — | — | — | — |
| FDSR | 0.20 | 0.80 | 0.52 | 0.43 | 0.78 | 0.43 | 0.34 | 0.51 | 0.00 | — | — | — | — | — | — | — | — | — | — | — | — | — | — | — | — | — | — | — |
| FDSS | 0.84 | 1.44 | 0.25 | 1.03 | 1.03 | 1.10 | 1.01 | 1.23 | 0.51 | 0.00 | — | — | — | — | — | — | — | — | — | — | — | — | — | — | — | — | — | — |
| FDPI | 0.22 | 0.77 | 0.62 | 0.35 | 0.73 | 0.39 | 0.34 | 0.43 | 0.34 | 0.73 | 0.00 | — | — | — | — | — | — | — | — | — | — | — | — | — | — | — | — | — |
| FDPM | 0.46 | 0.51 | 1.02 | 0.49 | 1.02 | 0.31 | 0.30 | 0.14 | 0.12 | 0.82 | 0.45 | 0.00 | — | — | — | — | — | — | — | — | — | — | — | — | — | — | — | — |
| FDPR | 0.24 | 0.63 | 0.71 | 0.50 | 0.95 | 0.32 | 0.08 | 0.38 | 0.52 | 1.25 | 0.30 | 0.33 | 0.00 | — | — | — | — | — | — | — | — | — | — | — | — | — | — | — |
| FDPS | 0.27 | 0.66 | 0.79 | 0.23 | 0.78 | 0.29 | 0.37 | 0.28 | 0.26 | 0.95 | 0.32 | 0.34 | 0.32 | 0.00 | — | — | — | — | — | — | — | — | — | — | — | — | — | — |
| FPL | 0.15 | 0.61 | 0.65 | 0.44 | 1.07 | 0.30 | 0.39 | 0.50 | 0.29 | 0.99 | 0.18 | 0.54 | 0.32 | 0.40 | 0.00 | — | — | — | — | — | — | — | — | — | — | — | — | — |
| EDCI | 0.77 | 1.38 | 0.20 | 0.96 | 1.03 | 0.91 | 0.37 | 1.13 | 0.63 | 0.21 | 0.36 | 1.14 | 0.84 | 0.88 | 0.81 | 0.03 | — | — | — | — | — | — | — | — | — | — | — | — |
| EDCM | 0.59 | 1.21 | 0.28 | 0.73 | 0.68 | 0.84 | 0.74 | 0.92 | 0.43 | 0.40 | 0.49 | 0.93 | 0.67 | 0.65 | 0.65 | 0.27 | 0.00 | — | — | — | — | — | — | — | — | — | — | — |
| EDCR | 0.58 | 1.20 | 0.10 | 0.80 | 0.87 | 0.85 | 0.75 | 0.97 | 0.46 | 0.27 | 0.56 | 0.98 | 0.68 | 0.73 | 0.61 | 0.22 | 0.20 | 0.00 | — | — | — | — | — | — | — | — | — | — |
| EDCS | 0.78 | 1.39 | 0.16 | 1.01 | 0.98 | 1.05 | 0.92 | 1.17 | 0.66 | 0.15 | 0.76 | 1.17 | 0.86 | 0.93 | 0.80 | 0.12 | 0.34 | 0.21 | 0.00 | — | — | — | — | — | — | — | — | — |
| EDQ | 0.61 | 1.19 | 0.12 | 0.89 | 1.01 | 0.87 | 0.72 | 1.00 | 0.51 | 0.34 | 0.62 | 0.99 | 0.67 | 0.79 | 0.62 | 0.30 | 0.36 | 0.20 | 0.24 | 0.00 | — | — | — | — | — | — | — | — |
| EIP | 0.77 | 1.39 | 0.20 | 0.91 | 1.04 | 0.79 | 0.94 | 1.15 | 0.65 | 0.12 | 0.74 | 1.17 | 0.87 | 0.90 | 0.80 | 0.12 | 0.28 | 0.20 | 0.12 | 0.31 | 0.00 | — | — | — | — | — | — | — |
| EPL | 0.53 | 1.11 | 0.19 | 0.79 | 1.04 | 0.79 | 0.72 | 0.95 | 0.48 | 0.35 | 0.58 | 0.96 | 0.65 | 0.74 | 0.51 | 0.39 | 0.38 | 0.21 | 0.32 | 0.19 | 0.34 | 0.00 | — | — | — | — | — | — |
| PT | 0.71 | 0.57 | 1.26 | 0.45 | 1.24 | 0.54 | 0.87 | 0.58 | 0.84 | 1.41 | 0.77 | 0.72 | 0.83 | 0.63 | 0.72 | 1.38 | 1.15 | 1.19 | 1.39 | 1.27 | 1.34 | 1.15 | 0.00 | — | — | — | — | — |
| PQ | 0.92 | 1.42 | 0.75 | 0.87 | 0.86 | 1.10 | 1.18 | 1.20 | 0.86 | 0.69 | 0.87 | 1.28 | 1.11 | 0.95 | 0.95 | 0.72 | 0.62 | 0.68 | 0.76 | 0.86 | 0.64 | 0.77 | 1.14 | 0.00 | — | — | — | — |
| BR | 1.03 | 1.30 | 1.24 | 0.86 | 0.74 | 1.05 | 0.86 | 0.89 | 0.91 | 1.43 | 0.84 | 0.82 | 0.88 | 0.84 | 1.16 | 1.24 | 1.06 | 1.19 | 1.32 | 1.23 | 1.31 | 1.30 | 1.34 | 1.48 | 0.00 | — | — | — |
| FDS | 2.32 | 1.93 | 2.91 | 2.48 | 2.06 | 2.08 | 2.28 | 1.93 | 2.41 | 3.08 | 2.30 | 1.98 | 2.30 | 2.13 | 2.37 | 3.01 | 2.75 | 2.84 | 3.05 | 2.91 | 3.00 | 2.83 | 1.80 | 2.77 | 2.26 | 0.00 | — | — |
| FDP | 3.30 | 2.89 | 3.89 | 3.42 | 3.04 | 3.06 | 3.25 | 2.91 | 3.39 | 4.06 | 3.28 | 2.95 | 3.27 | 3.10 | 3.35 | 3.98 | 3.72 | 3.82 | 4.03 | 3.89 | 3.98 | 3.81 | 2.77 | 3.73 | 3.16 | 0.98 | 0.00 | — |
| EDC | 0.54 | 0.76 | 1.02 | 0.77 | 0.23 | 0.48 | 0.66 | 0.41 | 0.56 | 1.17 | 0.45 | 0.52 | 0.62 | 0.31 | 0.65 | 1.09 | 0.83 | 0.93 | 1.14 | 1.04 | 1.08 | 0.97 | 0.50 | 0.94 | 0.91 | 1.92 | 2.90 | 0.00 |

Each muscle distal to the elbow is individually compared with all other muscles in terms of architecture. Lower values represent more similar muscles, and may guide surgeons in appropriate donor muscle selection by matching architectural properties, among several other considerations.

*Abbreviations:* EDCI, EDC index finger; EDCM, EDC middle finger; EDCR, EDC ring finger; EDCS, EDC small finger; FDSI/FDPI, FDS/FDP index finger; FDSM/FDPM, FDS/FDP middle finger; FDSR/FDPR, FDS/FDP ring finger; FDSS/FDPS, FDS/FDP small finger.

*From* Lieber RL, Jacobson MD, Fazeli BM, et al. Architecture of selected muscles of the arm and forearm: anatomy and implications for tendon transfer. J Hand Surg Am 1992;17(5):787–98; with permission.

and will be reasonably mobile due to the nature of fat. Brand[2] advocated using a blunt-headed tendon passer to gently create a path for a transferred tendon, as this would not damage the relatively immobile bony and fascial structures that the tendon passes; scarring to these caused by aggressive dissection would cause immediate failure.

The position of postoperative immobilization also determines final resistance. No matter how cautiously surgery is performed, adherence to local tissues is unavoidable. If these local tissues are reasonably mobile, they will allow some movement in both directions, although not without limit. To take advantage of this situation, the joint should be immobilized during healing in the middle of the expected range of motion to allow motion in both directions.[2] Immobilization at either of the extremes would only allow a small amount of motion in the opposite direction and should be avoided. Newer tendon coaptation techniques and hand therapy protocols have allowed earlier protected motion to limit adhesion formation, both in the field of tendon repair as well as tendon transfer.

### Tensioning

One area that remains poorly understood is that of how to appropriately tension a transferred tendon. Anecdotally, surgeons have for many years stated that tendons sewn in at higher tensions have functioned better. Part of the rationale for this is the observation that coaptations often lose tension with time, and this is believed to be counteracted by overtightening at the time of transfer. Further, many have observed that undertensioned muscles do not effectively contract after tendon transfer. These subjective observations have resulted in tendons being preferentially transferred at higher tension.

Much research over the past 30 years has focused on the relationship of passive tension to sarcomere length in an effort to make this process more objective. After all, muscles are transferred so as to provide muscle contraction in a deficient area rather than simply passive tension. Sarcomere length is the primary determinant of force generation, and although it is certainly related to the passive tension placed on a tendon intraoperatively, the correlation is not known at this time. In other words, surgeons placing passive tension on the transferred tendon cannot feel where on the Blix curve they are placing the tendon.[10]

For years, it was believed that all muscles adapted to chronic length changes by adding more sarcomeres in series to restore previous resting tension, based on studies in the soleus muscles of cats and rats.[11] More recent work by Friden and colleagues[12] in rabbit flexor digitorum longus (FDL) tendons showed that when sarcomere length was increased with a transfer, the response of the muscle over time was actually to decrease the number of serial sarcomeres, a stark contrast from earlier studies. Takahashi and colleagues[13] examined the effect of overtensioning a transferred tendon as measured by sarcomere length at the time of transfer. They found that the overtensioned muscle initially responded with an increase in serial sarcomeres, which dropped back to normal levels by 8 weeks. They also discovered a serial lengthening in the tendon, which occurred later than sarcomeric adaptation and was mediated by collagen catabolism as indicated by upregulated matrix metalloproteinases. Although these 2 animal studies are not directly transferrable to humans, they do cast doubt on previously held beliefs about tension equilibration and suggest a much more complex interplay of tendon tension, sarcomere generation, and tendon length.

Further studies have explored the important relationship between sarcomere length and intraoperative tension using laser diffraction methods. In 1985, Fleeter and colleagues[14] examined sarcomere length in cadaver arms after tendon transfer of flexor carpi ulnaris (FCU) to extensor digitorum communis (EDC) and palmaris longus (PL) to EPL, and noted them to be longer than optimal sarcomere length. They went on to use the same technique in 2 live patients undergoing the same transfer for radial nerve palsy. They found that after tensioning to the surgeons' best clinical judgment, the sarcomeres were longer than optimal. Lieber and colleagues[15] studied sarcomere length changes in FCU to EDC transfers using laser diffraction in 5 patients, noting that although sarcomere length increased, it did not reach the threshold they had calculated a priori to give the greatest tension from the FCU. Friden and Lieber[16] examined 22 patients undergoing various tendon transfers in the upper extremity. Transfers were performed by traditional passive tensioning by the surgeon to restore natural finger and wrist position. Sarcomere lengths were then determined with diffraction and compared with what had previously been calculated as optimal, and found uniformly to be excessively long, 3.78 μm on average compared with an ideal value of 2.8 μm. They concluded that muscles at that length could generate only approximately 28% of the maximal contraction for the muscles in question (**Fig. 5**).

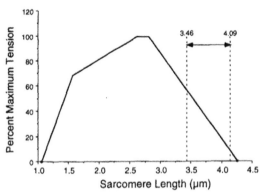

**Fig. 5.** When sarcomere length is measured after passive tensioning of a transferred tendon according to surgeon judgment, the length is found to be well outside of the optimal range for force generation. (*Adapted from* Friden J, Lieber RL. Evidence for muscle attachment at relatively long lengths in tendon transfer surgery. J Hand Surg Am 1998;23(1):105–10. 106; with permission.)

Although the feasibility of intraoperative laser diffraction limits broader application of this powerful technique, the findings of the previously discussed studies suggest that overtensioning a tendon at the time of transfer may at best reduce the maximum tension achievable by the muscle in question, and at worst, turn the procedure into a simple passive tenodesis.

## BIOMECHANICAL CHALLENGES
### *One Muscle Controlling Multiple Joints in Parallel*

Frequently in the setting of significant paralysis, numerous deficits are present with only a limited number of muscles available to replace them. As Brand[2] eloquently pointed out, it is not wise to be too ambitious in these settings, as attempting

to restore all the lost function would require single muscles to perform multiple functions, which limits the effectiveness of the transfer. This is due to the limitations of using a single motor with one excursion length to replace several previously independent muscles with differing excursions. By linking several insertions to the same tendon, as in the case of using 1 motor to restore metacarpophalangeal (MCP) flexion at all 4 fingers, the insertions will all move simultaneously. Further, the insertion with the shortest excursion will reach its maximally displaced position first and stop further motion of the muscle unit, thereby preventing full excursion at the remaining insertions (**Fig. 6**). These problems cannot be avoided, but by acknowledging them, care can be taken to limit their negative effects, by setting all insertions to a similar excursion, for example. Brand[2] advocated a deliberate approach to such cases, with extensive planning and intraoperative trialing of a transfer using temporary sutures before undertaking the definitive transfer.

### *One Muscle Controlling Multiple Joints in Series*

Another common scenario is that of the loss of intrinsic function following an ulnar nerve palsy. The sole remaining flexor of the thumb is the flexor pollicis longus (FPL). In the absence of a force, motion is excellent. However, in the setting of a distally applied force such as with a pinch maneuver, there is no support from more proximal flexors. Extensor torque is increased greatly at more proximal joints due to the longer lever arm there, and the thumb's only recourse to stabilize the joint is to flex the interphalangeal (IP) joint. This adds the same tension along the course of the tendon, so the force required to stabilize the MCP joint is also applied across the IP joint, which is far more than what is necessary,

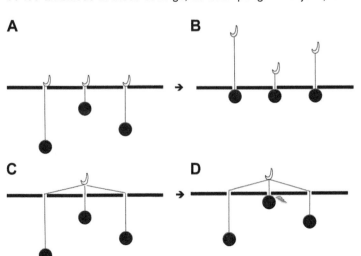

**A**

**B**

**C**

**D**

**Fig. 6.** Graphic depiction of transferring one muscle to multiple insertions. (*A*) Three weights are hung through a ceiling and attached to 3 independent hooks. (*B*) The hooks raise the weights until they reach the ceiling, preventing further movement. With independent hooks, each weight is moved through its entire range. (*C*) The 3 weights have now been transferred to a single hook, analogous to transferring 1 muscle to multiple insertions in parallel. (*D*) As the single hook raises the 3 weights, the middle weight with the shortest rope reaches full excursion first, preventing the other weights from being fully raised.

and hyperflexion results (**Fig. 7**). The solution to this problem is either to add independent flexors of the MCP joint or to fuse that joint, so that the FPL can appropriately regulate tension at the IP joint.[2]

## COAPTATION TECHNIQUES

The Pulvertaft (PT) weave has long been the standard coaptation technique in tendon transfers. One tendon end is weaved through the other in orthogonal passes, which are then secured with sutures. This has proven to be strong but is bulky, requires moderate length of available tendon, and remains susceptible to stripping given the linear orientation of collagen fibers. These disadvantages prompted a search for superior coaptation methods. This is particularly relevant as newer therapy protocols advocate for earlier motion to prevent adhesions and to orient healing collagen fibrils; solid tendon fixation at the time of surgery is essential to allowing this earlier motion.

Various alternative methods have been explored. The side-by-side (SS) coaptation requires little extra tendon and is relatively straightforward (**Fig. 8**A). Brown and colleagues[17] advocated a modified technique and found greater tensile strength to failure of SS as compared with PT secured with mattress stitches in cadaver tendons, as well as a stiffer repair. Bidic and colleagues[18] put forth a lasso technique, which when tested in porcine flexor tendons, was found to be equal in absolute strength to PT, with less time required to secure the coaptation and 7 fewer millimeters of tendon required. It was 5 mm thicker than PT on average, however, limiting appropriate anatomic locations (**Fig. 8**B). This finding was similar to the case of the double loop technique evaluated by Jeon and colleagues[19] They found strength to be increased compared with an end weave during the first 3 weeks, with equilibration of the 2 by week 4 (**Fig. 8**C). The investigators recommended this bulkier coaptation be used only on the dorsum of

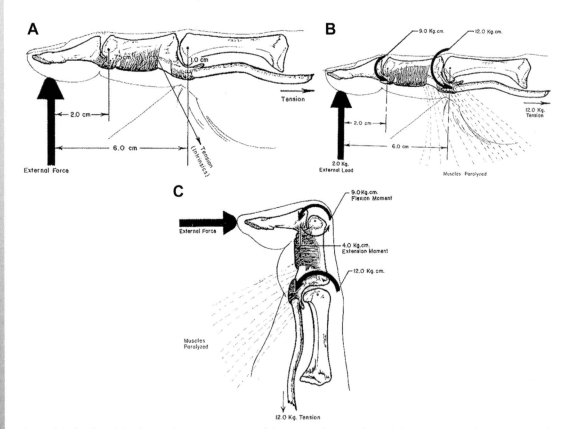

**Fig. 7.** (*A*) The thumb in ulnar palsy. Moment arms of the FPL at the IP and MCP joints are 0.75 and 1.0, respectively. The external load of 2.0 kg has a 2.0-cm moment arm at the IP joint and needs a flexor moment of 4.0 kg-cm for equilibrium. (*B*) For equilibrium at the MCP joint, a 2-kg load on the thumb pulp needs a 12.0-kg tension in the FPL tendon if other muscles are paralyzed. (*C*) The 12.0 kg tension that is needed to stabilize the MCP is much too great at the IP joint, and the latter goes into sharp flexion. (*Adapted from* Brand PW, Hollister A. Clinical mechanics of the hand. Second edition. St Louis (MO): Mosby Year Book; 1993. p. 85; with permission.)

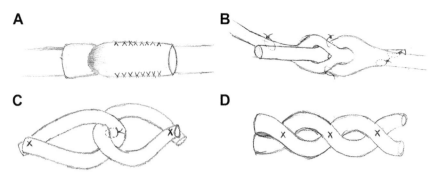

**Fig. 8.** (*A*) Side-to-side tenorrhaphy. The tendon is passed through a slit in the other tendon and then secured side-to-side with cross-stitches. (*B*) Modified Lasso technique. (*C*) Double loop technique. (*D*) Spiral technique.

the hand or in the forearm. Finally, Kulikov and colleagues[20] compared the spiral weave to the PT weave. They found absolute strength and profile to be essentially equivalent and advocated this method given its simplicity (**Fig. 8**D).

Although each method has advantages and disadvantages, most of these studies demonstrate equivalency with the PT weave. Assuming the bulkier methods are not used in finer settings, the wisest selection for the surgeon is likely that which he or she can reliably perform. Various suture techniques will also play a role in the overall strength of the transfer construct. Although an in-depth exploration of these is beyond the scope of this article, multiple studies have shown vertical mattress sutures to be inferior in both SS and PT techniques.[21,22]

## SUMMARY

The fundamental mechanics of tendon transfers are largely unchanged from the principles set forth by the earliest pioneers in the field. Many of the principles and challenges remain the same. However, a more nuanced understanding of sarcomere biology has brought better understanding of the influence of intraoperative passive tensioning on final muscle function, although it remains very challenging to confidently place the transferred tendon at a functionally advantageous sarcomere length. New tendon coaptation methods provide further options to the surgeon, allowing a more versatile approach.

## REFERENCES

1. Brand PW, Hollister A. Clinical mechanics of the hand. Second edition. St Louis (MO): Mosby Year Book; 1993.
2. Brand P. Biomechanics of tendon transfers. In: Burkhalter W, editor. Hand clinics: tendon transfers, vol. 4. Philadelphia: W.B. Saunders Company; 1988. p. 137–54.
3. Walker SM, Schrodt GR. I segment lengths and thin filament periods in skeletal muscle fibers of the Rhesus monkey and the human. Anat Rec 1974;178(1):63–81.
4. Brand PW, Beach MA, Thompson DE. Relative tension and potential excursion of muscles in the forearm and hand. J Hand Surg 1981;6(3):209–19.
5. Granzier H, Labeit S. Structure-function relations of the giant elastic protein titin in striated and smooth muscle cells. Muscle Nerve 2007;36(6):740–55.
6. Boyes JH. Selection of a donor muscle for tendon transfer. Bull Hosp Joint Dis 1962;23:1–4.
7. Friden J, Ward SR, Smallwood L, et al. Passive muscle-tendon amplitude may not reflect skeletal muscle functional excursion. J Hand Surg Am 2006;31(7):1105–10.
8. Lieber RL, Jacobson MD, Fazeli BM, et al. Architecture of selected muscles of the arm and forearm: anatomy and implications for tendon transfer. J Hand Surg Am 1992;17(5):787–98.
9. Bunnell S. Hand surgery. J Bone Joint Surg Am 1947;29(3):824.
10. Lieber RL. Biology and mechanics of skeletal muscle: what hand surgeons need to know when tensioning a tendon transfer. J Hand Surg Am 2008;33(9):1655–6.
11. Baker JH, Hall-Craggs EC. Changes in length of sarcomeres following tenotomy of the rat soleus muscle. Anat Rec 1978;192(1):55–8.
12. Friden J, Ponten E, Lieber RL. Effect of muscle tension during tendon transfer on sarcomerogenesis in a rabbit model. J Hand Surg Am 2000;25(1):138–43.
13. Takahashi M, Ward SR, Marchuk LL, et al. Asynchronous muscle and tendon adaptation after surgical tensioning procedures. J Bone Joint Surg Am 2010;92(3):664–74.
14. Fleeter TB, Adams JP, Brenner B, et al. A laser diffraction method for measuring muscle sarcomere length in vivo for application to tendon transfers. J Hand Surg Am 1985;10(4):542–6.
15. Lieber RL, Ponten E, Burkholder TJ, et al. Sarcomere length changes after flexor carpi ulnaris to extensor digitorum communis tendon transfer. J Hand Surg Am 1996;21(4):612–8.

16. Friden J, Lieber RL. Evidence for muscle attachment at relatively long lengths in tendon transfer surgery. J Hand Surg Am 1998;23(1): 105–10.

17. Brown SH, Hentzen ER, Kwan A, et al. Mechanical strength of the side-to-side versus Pulvertaft weave tendon repair. J Hand Surg Am 2010; 35(4):540–5.

18. Bidic SM, Varshney A, Ruff MD, et al. Biomechanical comparison of lasso, Pulvertaft weave, and side-by-side tendon repairs. Plast Reconstr Surg 2009;124(2):567–71.

19. Jeon SH, Chung MS, Baek GH, et al. Comparison of loop-tendon versus end-weave methods for tendon transfer or grafting in rabbits. J Hand Surg Am 2009;34(6):1074–9.

20. Kulikov YI, Dodd S, Gheduzzi S, et al. An in vitro biomechanical study comparing the spiral linking technique against the Pulvertaft weave for tendon repair. J Hand Surg Eur Vol 2007;32(4):377–81.

21. Wagner E, Ortiz C, Wagner P, et al. Biomechanical evaluation of various suture configurations in side-to-side tenorrhaphy. J Bone Joint Surg Am 2014;96(3):232–6.

22. Tanaka T, Zhao C, Ettema AM, et al. Tensile strength of a new suture for fixation of tendon grafts when using a weave technique. J Hand Surg Am 2006; 31(6):982–6.

# Restoration of Shoulder Function

Chelsea C. Boe, MD[a],*, Bassem T. Elhassan, MD[b]

## KEYWORDS

- Tendon transfer • External rotation • Brachial plexus injury • Lower trapezius
- Global shoulder dysfunction

## KEY POINTS

- Surgical management of shoulder paralysis after brachial plexus injury requires multispecialty approach.
- Restoration of external rotation is a priority following paralyzing injury.
- Lower trapezius transfer is a reliable procedure for restoration of external rotation.
- Multiple tendon transfers about the shoulder are utilized to restore global shoulder function provide optimal outcomes.

## INTRODUCTION

Brachial plexus injury, although rare, represents a severe and life-altering injury with a variable degree of shoulder and arm dysfunction. Paralysis of the deltoid and rotator cuff muscles results in loss of abduction, external rotation as well as potentially painful inferior glenohumeral subluxation.[1–3] Because of the predominance of upper trunk injuries and innervation pattern through the plexus, the deltoid and rotator cuff are involved in 91% and 100% of palsies, respectively.[4]

Brachial plexus nerve reconstruction, with or without free muscle transfer, has been reported to lead to a good outcome in restoring elbow function in most cases.[2] However, restoration of shoulder motion, namely external rotation, has been disappointing.[3,5] Suzuki and colleagues[1] demonstrated that, at a mean follow-up of 28 months after neurotization of the suprascapular nerve from the spinal accessory nerve, external rotation was only 16.7°. Bertelli and Ghizoni[3] noted no return of external rotation after complete brachial

plexus palsy treated with transfer of the spinal accessory to suprascapular nerve.

Historical treatment of shoulder paralysis involved arthrodesis of the glenohumeral joint for stability. However, function was reliant on scapulothoracic motion, which could be compromised in this patient population, especially in those with compromised trapezius muscle after spinal accessory nerve transfer,[6–8] which has led previous investigators to recommend arthrodesis as a salvage procedure for a paralyzed shoulder when alternate attempts at functional restoration have failed.[9–12] The authors advocate for the use of tendon transfers as the preferred treatment modality for patients with shoulder paralysis.

The complex motion of the shoulder in multiple planes requires smooth synergy of primary movers and stabilizers of both the glenohumeral and the scapulothoracic articulations. Knowledge of the anatomy and complex interplay of opposing muscle groups in cooperating joints is necessary to focus reconstructive efforts and identify acceptable tendons to sacrifice for transfer. General principles of transfer include targeting muscles with

The authors have nothing to disclose.
[a] Department of Orthopedic Surgery, Mayo Clinic, 200 1st Street Southwest, Rochester, MN 55905, USA;
[b] Department of Orthopedic Surgery, College of Medicine, Mayo Clinic, 200 1st Street Southwest, Rochester, MN 55905, USA
* Corresponding author.
*E-mail address:* Boe.Chelsea@mayo.edu

similar excursion and tension, expendability, at least M4 strength, and a similar line of pull to the nonfunctional muscle. The transferred muscle should also be used for a single purpose.[13]

Early attempts at tendon transfers to address shoulder dysfunction following nerve injury emphasized restoration of abduction and flexion. Historically described transfers include the upper trapezius to the proximal humerus, first described in 1891 by Hoffa, later by Lewis in 1910 and Lange in 1911,[11] and ultimately modified by Saha, whose name is now associated with this surgery.[9] However, recovery of abduction and flexion was limited with this transfer, resulting in persistent dysfunction and a largely useless extremity[4,14]; this was partially attributed to the shorter lever arm of the upper trapezius as well as the resection of acromion, which allowed for superior escape of the humeral head. Pedicled latissimus transfer for restoration of the abduction and forward flexion after deltoid paralysis has been described by Itoh and colleagues.[15] Although results were promising in patients with intact rotator cuff musculature, they were less impressive in the setting of paralyzed rotator cuff muscles, leading to the recommendation that rotator cuff muscle reconstruction should be used in conjunction with attempts at restoration of abduction and/or forward flexion.[15] The appreciation of the need to address the stabilizing musculature of the shoulder for improved functional recovery was actually advocated in the earlier recommendations for multiple tendon transfers by Saha, although colloquially associated with the isolated upper trapezius transfer.[9]

Rotator cuff muscle dysfunction contributes to poorer results in flexion and abduction given their contribution to those motions as stabilizers of the joint to maintain appropriate humeral contact with the glenoid. Improved understanding of the need for stability of the joint in addition to primary mobilizers for flexion, abduction, and external rotations guides priorities in secondary repair after global shoulder injury. It should also be appreciated that in addition to the potential for rotator cuff denervation, rotator cuff tears can occur in up to 10% of cases.[16]

Besides to stabilization of the glenohumeral joint, one of the most important functions of the rotator cuff is shoulder external rotation. The significance of external rotation in performing activities of daily living (ADLs) has been identified. In fact, most ADLs are performed with some degree of external rotation with the arm positioned with only 27° of abduction most of the time.[17] Langer and colleagues[18] found that limitation in external rotation significantly impaired ADLs and

concluded that even modest improvement in external rotation in the setting of complete paralysis would greatly improve competency and independence in ADLs.

Obligate internal rotation, despite restored elbow flexion, results in a "hand-on-belly" position.[2,19] According to the grading system by Doi and colleagues,[20] the lack of ability to stabilize the shoulder joint and position the hand in space represents an outcome classified as less than poor.

Anatomic, functional, and biomechanical studies have been conducted to determine the relative contributions of individual rotator cuff muscles to shoulder function. Subscapularis contributes 52% to the abduction moment arm as calculated by multiplying cross-sectional area by lever arm.[21] Infraspinatus and teres minor collectively represent 45% of the external rotation moment arm, whereas subscapularis contributes 42% of internal rotation by a similar estimation.[21] These measurements were correlated with clinical evaluation using nerve blocks. Paralysis of the infraspinatus alone led to 70% loss of abduction strength, whereas paralysis of both supraspinatus and infraspinatus led to approximately 75% loss of abduction strength and 80% of external rotation strength.[22] These findings support targeting restoration of the infraspinatus function to maximize external rotation with a single tendon transfer.

Previously described tendon transfers using the latissimus dorsi and/or teres major to restore external rotation in upper plexus palsy should be considered contraindicated in global injury. Because of their line of pull and absent deltoid function, these may in fact lead to worsening inferior subluxation.[9] In addition, these muscles could be affected in the paralytic shoulder, depending on the extent of the injury. On the other hand, the function of the trapezius, levator scapulae, and rhomboids is preserved or recovered in 96% of cases of brachial plexus palsy,[12] representing consistently viable options for tendon transfer in an otherwise limited setting. Herzberg and colleagues[23] demonstrated the potential for division of multipennate muscles into functional subcomponents, further expanding the armamentarium of available transfers. Although these divisions have been demonstrated to be independently significant scapula stabilizers in the athlete,[24] normal function of other scapula stabilizers seems to be protective of dysfunction on harvest of subcomponents.[19]

Elhassan and colleagues[19] described lower trapezius transfer to reconstruct shoulder external rotation in patients with brachial plexus injury and reported successful outcome in most patients.[25]

A well-designed biomechanical study performed by Hartzler and colleagues[26] showed a significantly better moment arm of external rotation of the lower trapezius transfer when compared with the latissimus or teres major transfer.[19,25] When lower trapezius is deficient, generally as a result of prior spinal accessory nerve transfer, the contralateral lower trapezius has been shown to be feasible for transfer to reconstruct shoulder external rotation.[27,28]

In the senior author's practice, when planning to improve shoulder function in patients with brachial plexus injury, the priority is to attempt restoration of shoulder stability and external rotation function. If, in addition to the trapezius, periscapular muscles (mainly pectoralis major and latissimus dorsi) are available with at least grade 4 strength, then additional transfers could be performed to further improve shoulder motion.[29,30] In this review, the authors focus on transfer of the different parts of the trapezius, which is the more common and standard transfer in patients with traumatic brachial plexus injury.

### Preoperative Planning

Initial evaluation of a paralyzed shoulder involves a complete history and physical examination with specific attention to the remaining function of surrounding muscles and identification of deficits that detract significantly from quality of life and ability to perform ADLs. Specifically, this entails clinical assessment of subluxation, degree of active motion of each independent muscle around the shoulder as well as shoulder stiffness and integrity of scapula stabilizers. It is important to have a thorough understanding of previous procedures and attempts at primary repair, because this may alter innervation and thus available tendons for transfer. Radiographs are obtained to assess for implants, fracture, glenohumeral arthritis, and subluxation. The precise treatment plan is tailored to the specific patient based on synthesis of this information with the previously detailed goals in mind. The authors' preference is to transfer the lower trapezius to the infraspinatus tendon to restore shoulder external rotation, and the upper/middle trapezius to the proximal humerus to stabilize and reduce the shoulder from inferior subluxation as well as marginally improve shoulder flexion/abduction. If latissimus and pectoralis major are available, then either of these muscles could be transferred as a pedicled flap to reconstruct the anterior deltoid for shoulder flexion.

### SURGICAL TECHNIQUE
#### Preparation and Patient Positioning

The surgical technique for lower trapezius transfer has been previously reported,[19,25] as has the

authors' technique for multiple transfers to restore global function of the shoulder.[29]

Standard positioning is lateral with the operative side up (the uninvolved shoulder can be prepared into the field if needed for contralateral lower trapezius transfer, although for this description, the authors will presume ipsilateral lower trapezius is available). All bony prominences are well padded. Nerve stimulation can be used intraoperatively to address any concerns about viability of innervation to muscles for transfer.

### Surgical Approach and Procedure

If isolated lower trapezius transfer is performed, the authors perform an incision medial to the scapula and an additional inverted L-incision laterally at the level of the palpable glenohumeral joint (**Fig. 1**). The details of harvesting of the lower trapezius and passing to attach it to the infraspinatus tendon are very similar in this technique to the more extensile technique reported in later discussion. The main differences are the incisions performed and creation of tunnel between the medial and lateral wound to pass the trapezius tendon from medial to lateral (**Fig. 2**).

The authors' standard extensile approach when performing multiple tendon transfers around the shoulder is an inverted U-shaped incision, beginning medial to the scapula, distal to the medial spine, and extending proximally and laterally toward the acromion and then distally to the level of the mid deltoid (**Fig. 3**). Skin flaps are elevated,

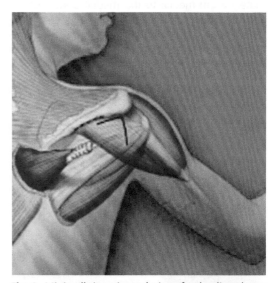

**Fig. 1.** Minimally invasive technique for the direct lower trapezius transfer to the infraspinatus through double incision technique. (*Courtesy of* Mayo Foundation for Medical Education and Research, Rochester, MN; with permission.)

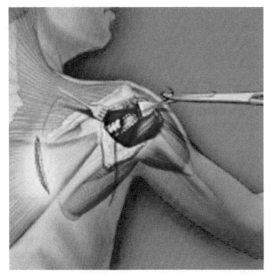

**Fig. 2.** Lower trapezius passed from medial incision to lateral incision through deep tunnel and directly attached to the infraspinatus tendon. (*Courtesy of* Mayo Foundation for Medical Education and Research, Rochester, MN; with permission.)

and the trapezius muscle is identified (**Fig. 4**). The lateral aspect of the lower trapezius is dissected and followed to the medial spine of the scapula, where the tendinous insertion of the lower trapezius is detached. The interval between the lower and middle trapezius is developed and dissected to separate these 2 portions of the trapezius muscle. The spinal accessory nerve is identified deep in the dissection field, approximately 2 cm medial to the medial border of the scapula. The deep location of the nerve on the undersurface of the muscle allows for safe separation of the muscle fibers of the middle and lower trapezius (**Fig. 5**). Once adequately mobilized, 2

number 2 nonabsorbable sutures are placed in Krakow fashion in the lower trapezius tendon to prepare it for transfer. The lower trapezius muscle and tendon are temporarily placed in the wound to prevent desiccation.

Attention is then directed toward the elevation and preparation of the rest of the trapezius for transfer. The authors previously reported the transfer of the upper/middle trapezius with their acromial bony attachment to the humerus.[19] Although excellent fixation of the transfer to the proximal humerus and good stability of the shoulder were achieved with this technique, the gain of function was minimal. The authors think that this is related to the loss of the flexion/abduction moment arm of the transferred trapezius. For this reason, they have modified their technique by performing an osteotomy of the lateral 5 to 10 mm of the lateral acromion while retaining the trapezius insertion (**Fig. 6**). The transfer is performed by passing it over the remaining acromion and attaching it to the proximal humerus distal to the greater tuberosity. This modification has 2 main advantages: improvement of the moment arm of flexion/abduction of the transferred trapezius and allowance for better distal reach of the transfer by shortening of the acromion.

The authors start the sequence of transfers with the lower trapezius transfer because it is easier to perform with the shoulder in adduction and maximal external rotation. This shoulder position would be difficult to attain if they performed the upper/middle trapezius transfer first.

The paralyzed posterior deltoid is detached. The infraspinatus tendon is dissected, and the length of the tendon obtained after adequate dissection is 4 to 7 cm. The tendon is tagged with double

**Fig. 3.** The authors' standard marking for the incision they perform for the exposure in multiple tendon transfers around the shoulder in patients with brachial plexus injury. (*Courtesy of* Mayo Foundation for Medical Education and Research, Rochester, MN; with permission.)

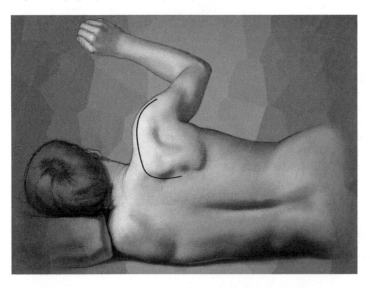

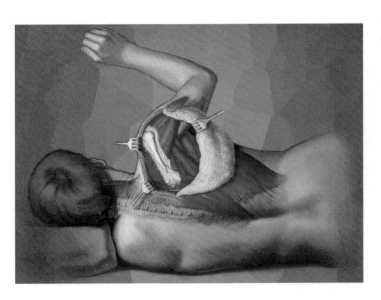

**Fig. 4.** The exposure achieved from the incision delineated in **Fig. 3**. (*Courtesy of* Mayo Foundation for Medical Education and Research, Rochester, MN; with permission.)

number 2 nonabsorbable sutures that are placed in Krakow fashion. Then, while keeping the shoulder adducted and in maximal external rotation, direct transfer of the lower trapezius tendon to the infraspinatus tendon is performed. The authors use the sutures that were previously placed in both tendons to perform the repair. They wrap the tendon transfer construct with TenoGlide (Integra Lifesciences, Plainsboro, NJ, USA) to decrease the risk of scarring along the track of the transfer.

The shoulder is then placed in 80° of abduction (this is modified to 60° of abduction in patients with prior free-muscle transfer to restore elbow flexion that has been innervated by intercostal nerves, to protect these nerves) to prepare it for the upper/middle trapezius transfer. The proximal-lateral humerus is debrided with electrical burr distal to the greater tuberosity. TenoGlide (Integra Lifesciences) is placed on top of the acromion, and the upper/middle trapezius is passed over the top of the acromion and inserted on the prepared proximal humerus (**Fig. 7**). Two 3.0 cannulated cancellous screws are used to secure the detached acromial segment on the proximal humerus. The authors reinforce the repair with multiple transosseous sutures that are passed through the tendinous insertion of the transferred trapezius. Then, the detached deltoid is partly reattached on the acromion and partly on the transferred trapezius.

### *Immediate Postoperative Care*

The shoulder is maintained in abduction and external rotation for 8 weeks after surgery by way of brace or spica cast. The suction drain is removed when the drainage is less than 30 mL in a 24-hour period. Patients are encouraged to keep the ipsilateral hand and contralateral shoulder mobile. The authors recommend against heavy lifting, pushing, or pulling with the contralateral hand for the first 2 months until the immobilization is discontinued.

### REHABILITATION AND RECOVERY

On completion of 8 weeks of strict abduction and external rotation postoperatively, progressive adduction of the extremity is allowed over the subsequent 2 weeks. Active-assisted range

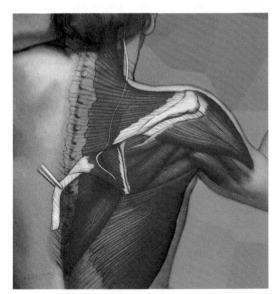

**Fig. 5.** Lower trapezius harvesting as preparation to transfer. (*Courtesy of* Mayo Foundation for Medical Education and Research, Rochester, MN; with permission.)

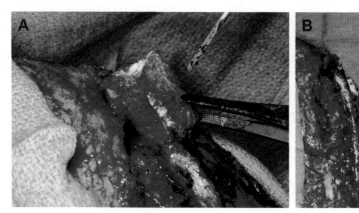

**Fig. 6.** (*A*, *B*) Upper and middle trapezius harvesting with 1 cm of acromial insertion while leaving the rest of the acromion intact.

of motion is performed for 6 weeks with aqua therapy, but no passive stretching is allowed; this is followed by active motion for 6 weeks, including swimming exercises. Strengthening is subsequently initiated, and the patient progresses to unrestricted activities at 6 months postoperatively.

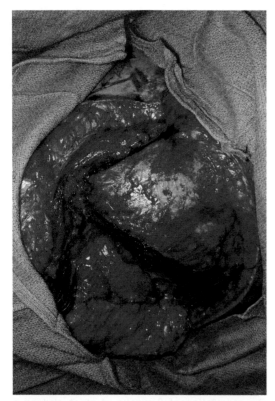

**Fig. 7.** The final look of the lower trapezius transfer to the infraspinatus tendon, and upper/middle trapezius transfer on top of the acromion onto the proximal humerus.

## CLINICAL RESULTS IN THE LITERATURE

The significant variability in individual cases makes direct comparison among patients and specific transfers difficult. Upper trapezius transfer in isolation has been frequently attempted with modest results in terms of global shoulder function. Aziz and colleagues[31] reported 40° improvement in flexion and abduction with the Saha[9] technique. Monreal and colleagues[32] published results of 10 patients after brachial plexus injury with average improvement of 40° abduction and flexion after trapezius transfer. This transfer was also noted to correct glenohumeral subluxation. Ruhmann and colleagues[4,14] have published their results with this procedure in brachial plexus injuries, noting improved outcomes for patients with functional biceps, coracobrachialis, pectoralis major, or triceps muscles. Patients with completely flailed shoulders gained 28° of abduction and 19° of flexion compared with 42° of abduction and 56° of flexion in those with incomplete nerve injuries. These results may be attributed to the stabilization of the glenohumeral joint with intact secondary musculature. They also reported a modification of the Saha technique incorporating the deltoid fibers on maximal tension to the transferred upper trapezius such that the force may be transmitted through the fibers of the deltoid, extending the lever arm and more closely approximating native anatomic abduction.[4,14]

None of these studies addressed or reported external rotation function in their patients and its contribution to overall shoulder function, which has been shown to have a significant effect on patient satisfaction and ability to perform ADLs.[18]

Elhassan and colleagues[19] originally reported the lower trapezius transfer in a patient who had no active external rotation preoperatively and showed significant improvement in shoulder external rotation. The same investigators subsequently reported on the outcome of multiple tendon transfers, including lower trapezius, and showed that the improvement in shoulder external rotation was reliable and achieved in more than 90% of patients; however, the improvement of shoulder abduction and flexion was only modest and not significant.[19,25,27,29,30] The senior author has performed more than 300 lower trapezius transfers, either isolated or in the setting of multiple tendon transfers for different shoulder disorders, and observed that this transfer is very reliable in restoring shoulder external rotation. For this reason, it is the tendon transfer of choice that is performed to regain shoulder external rotation in the authors' practice.

Bertelli and colleagues[33] describe a similar technique with transfer of upper trapezius to restore abduction and lower trapezius to the tendon of the infraspinatus in 7 patients with upper brachial plexus palsies. They reported an average increase of 38° of abduction and 104° of external rotation (as measured from full internal rotation).

When the ipsilateral trapezius is not available, the contralateral lower trapezius origin has been shown to be feasible for transfer to the ipsilateral infraspinatus tendon to restore shoulder external rotation.[27] Satbhai and colleagues[28] showed significant improvement in external rotation and reproducible improvement in functional scores in 3 patients, who underwent contralateral lower trapezius transfer. Similarly, Elhassan and colleagues[29] in a more recent study showed significant improvement in shoulder external rotation in 8 of 12 patients.

## SUMMARY

Reconstruction of shoulder function in adult patients with brachial plexus injury can be very challenging. The most common presenting symptoms are pain, inferior shoulder subluxation, and lack of shoulder function, notably external rotation, which is essential to position the hand in the space. When trapezius muscle is available for transfer, studies have shown that the lower trapezius transfer is reliable in improving shoulder external rotation, and upper/middle trapezius transfer is reliable in reducing inferior shoulder subluxation and improving associated pain. Further improvement in shoulder flexion is possible if latissimus or pectoralis muscles are available for transfer. Long-term studies should be performed to determine the longevity of these transfers over time.

## REFERENCES

1. Suzuki K, Doi K, Hattori Y, et al. Long-term results of spinal accessory nerve transfer to the suprascapular nerve in upper-type paralysis of brachial plexus injury. J Reconstr Microsurg 2007;23(6):295–9.
2. Shin AY, Spinner RJ, Steinmann SP, et al. Adult traumatic brachial plexus injuries. J Am Acad Orthop Surg 2005;13(6):382–96.
3. Bertelli JA, Ghizoni MF. Transfer of the accessory nerve to the suprascapular nerve in brachial plexus reconstruction. J Hand Surg 2007;32(7):989–98.
4. Ruhmann O, Schmolke S, Bohnsack M, et al. Trapezius transfer in brachial plexus palsy. Correlation of the outcome with muscle power and operative technique. J Bone Joint Surg Br 2005;87(2):184–90.
5. Doi K, Hattori Y, Ikeda K, et al. Significance of shoulder function in the reconstruction of prehension with double free-muscle transfer after complete paralysis of the brachial plexus. Plast Reconstr Surg 2003;112(6):1596–603.
6. Vastamaki M. Shoulder arthrodesis for paralysis and arthrosis. Acta Orthop Scand 1987;58(5):549–53.
7. Hawkins RJ, Neer CS 2nd. A functional analysis of shoulder fusion. Clin Orthop Relat Res 1987;(223): 65–76.
8. Cofield RH, Briggs BT. Glenohumeral arthrodesis. Operative and long-term functional results. J Bone Joint Surg Am 1979;61(5):668–77.
9. Saha AK. Surgery of the paralysed and flail shoulder. Acta Orthop Scand 1967;(Suppl 97):5–90.
10. Goldner JL. Strengthening of the partially paralyzed shoulder girdle by multiple muscle-tendon transfers. Hand Clin 1988;4(2):323–36.
11. Ruhmann O, Wirth CJ, Gossé F, et al. Trapezius transfer after brachial plexus palsy. Indications, difficulties and complications. J Bone Joint Surg Br 1998;80(1):109–13.
12. Narakas AO. Muscle transpositions in the shoulder and upper arm for sequelae of brachial plexus palsy. Clin Neurol Neurosurg 1993; 95(Suppl):S89–91.
13. Brand PW, Beach RB, Thompson DE. Relative tension and potential excursion of muscles in the forearm and hand. J Hand Surg 1981;6(3):209–19.
14. Ruhmann O, Schmolke S, Bohnsack M, et al. Reconstructive operations for the upper limb after brachial plexus palsy. Am J Orthop (Belle Mead NJ) 2004;33(7):351–62.
15. Itoh Y, Sasaki T, Ishiguro T, et al. Transfer of latissimus dorsi to replace a paralysed anterior deltoid. A new technique using an inverted pedicled graft. J Bone Joint Surg Br 1987;69(4):647–51.
16. Brogan DM, Carofino BC, Kircher MF, et al. Prevalence of rotator cuff tears in adults with traumatic brachial plexus injuries. J Bone Joint Surg Am 2014;96(16):e139.

17. Raiss P, Rettig O, Wolf S, et al. Range of motion of shoulder and elbow in activities of daily life in 3D motion analysis. Z Orthop Unfall 2007;145(4):493–8 [in German].

18. Langer JS, Sueoka SS, Wang AA. The importance of shoulder external rotation in activities of daily living: improving outcomes in traumatic brachial plexus palsy. J Hand Surg 2012;37(7):1430–6.

19. Elhassan B, Bishop A, Shin A. Trapezius transfer to restore external rotation in a patient with a brachial plexus injury. A case report. J Bone Joint Surg Am 2009;91(4):939–44.

20. Doi K, Muramatsu K, Hattori Y, et al. Restoration of prehension with the double free muscle technique following complete avulsion of the brachial plexus. Indications and long-term results. J Bone Joint Surg Am 2000;82(5):652–66.

21. Bassett RW, Browne AO, Morrey BF, et al. Glenohumeral muscle force and moment mechanics in a position of shoulder instability. J Biomech 1990; 23(5):405–15.

22. Gerber C, Blumenthal S, Curt A, et al. Effect of selective experimental suprascapular nerve block on abduction and external rotation strength of the shoulder. J Shoulder Elbow Surg 2007;16(6): 815–20.

23. Herzberg G, Urien JP, Dimnet J. Potential excursion and relative tension of muscles in the shoulder girdle: relevance to tendon transfers. J Shoulder Elbow Surg 1999;8(5):430–7.

24. Kibler WB, Chandler TJ, Shapiro R, et al. Muscle activation in coupled scapulohumeral motions in the high performance tennis serve. Br J Sports Med 2007;41(11):745–9.

25. Elhassan B. Lower trapezius transfer for shoulder external rotation in patients with paralytic shoulder. J Hand Surg 2014;39(3):556–62.

26. Hartzler RU, Barlow JD, An KN, et al. Biomechanical effectiveness of different types of tendon transfers to the shoulder for external rotation. J Shoulder Elbow Surg 2012;21(10):1370–6.

27. Elhassan BT, Wagner ER, Bishop AT. Feasibility of contralateral trapezius transfer to restore shoulder external rotation: part I. J Shoulder Elbow Surg 2012;21(10):1363–9.

28. Satbhai NG, Doi K, Hattori Y, et al. Contralateral lower trapezius transfer for restoration of shoulder external rotation in traumatic brachial plexus palsy: a preliminary report and literature review. J Hand Surg Eur Vol 2014;39(8):861–7.

29. Elhassan B, Bishop AT, Hartzler RU, et al. Tendon transfer options about the shoulder in patients with brachial plexus injury. J Bone Joint Surg Am 2012; 94(15):1391–8.

30. Elhassan B, Bishop A, Shin A, et al. Shoulder tendon transfer options for adult patients with brachial plexus injury. J Hand Surg Am 2010;35(7):1211–9.

31. Aziz W, Singer RM, Wolff TW. Transfer of the trapezius for flail shoulder after brachial plexus injury. J Bone Joint Surg Br 1990;72(4):701–4.

32. Monreal R, Paredes L, Diaz H, et al. Trapezius transfer to treat flail shoulder after brachial plexus palsy. J Brachial Plex Peripher Nerve Inj 2007;2:2.

33. Bertelli JA. Upper and lower trapezius muscle transfer to restore shoulder abduction and external rotation in longstanding upper type palsies of the brachial plexus in adults. Microsurgery 2011;31(4): 263–7.

# Restoration of Elbow Flexion

Bryan J. Loeffler, MD*, Daniel R. Lewis, MD

## KEYWORDS

- Elbow flexion • Tendon transfer • Latissimus dorsi • Pectoralis major • Triceps to biceps
- Steindler flexorplasty

## KEY POINTS

- The latissimus dorsi, pectoralis major, flexor-pronator mass, and triceps are all options when considering muscle transfer to restore elbow flexion, and a thorough preoperative assessment is required to determine the ideal transfer.
- The bipolar latissimus transfer produces the greatest strength and additionally can be performed as a myocutaneous flap to assist in soft tissue coverage.
- Pectoralis major transfer is reliable for restoring elbow flexion, but is the most cosmetically deforming option.
- Steindler flexorplasty produces weak elbow flexion, but reduces active supination and often requires concomitant wrist and digital flexion with elbow flexion, which can limit its functional advantage.
- Triceps to biceps transfer restores elbow flexion, but sacrifices active elbow extension and can produce significant elbow flexion contractures in the long term. Isolated long head of triceps transfer may allow for restoration of elbow flexion without sacrificing active elbow extension, but clinical results are limited.

## INTRODUCTION

The loss of active elbow flexion is disabling, particularly when the hand is functional. Several procedures have been described to restore elbow flexion, including unipolar or bipolar transfer of the pectoralis major, Steindler flexorplasty, unipolar or bipolar transfer of latissimus dorsi, triceps to biceps transfer, pectoralis minor transfer, and sternocleidomastoid transfer.

Loss of elbow flexion most commonly occurs following brachial plexus injury, proximal injury to the musculocutaneous nerve, or anterior elbow trauma, which results in irreparable damage to the biceps and brachialis. Arthrogryposis, particularly the amyoplasia form, is often associated with the inability to actively flex the elbow, but with preserved elbow extension. In addition, elbow flexion

paralysis was seen due to poliomyelitis infection historically. Patients with preserved hand and wrist function, but a lack of elbow flexion are limited by their inability to position the hand in space.

The principles of any tendon transfer must be followed when considering a transfer to restore elbow flexion. These include, but are not limited to, assessment of available muscle donors, including their work capacity and mechanical advantage, presence of passive elbow flexion, and potential disability created as a result of the transfer. In addition, matching the line of pull and excursion of the biceps is ideal for a transfer aimed at improving elbow flexion.

In the case of recent brachial plexus injury, patients may be candidates for nerve grafting or distal nerve transfers. If these procedures have been performed, it is recommended to wait 2 years

OrthoCarolina Hand Center, 1915 Randolph Road, Charlotte, NC 28207, USA
* Corresponding author.
*E-mail address:* Bryan.loeffler@orthocarolina.com

Hand Clin 32 (2016) 311–321
http://dx.doi.org/10.1016/j.hcl.2016.03.002
0749-0712/16/$ – see front matter © 2016 Elsevier Inc. All rights reserved.

postoperatively before determining that muscle transfer is required.

## TRANSFER OPTIONS
### Pectoralis Major Transfers

#### Introduction
Utilization of the pectoralis major to restore elbow flexion has been described and performed for almost a century. Procedures include pectoralis flexorplasty, unipolar and bipolar reconstructions, combined pectoralis minor and major transfers, and isolated pectoralis minor transfers.

#### Anatomy
The pectoralis major is composed of 2 anatomic components: the clavicular and sternocostal portions. The clavicular head originates from the medial clavicle and is innervated by the lateral pectoral nerve (C5–C7). It is nourished primarily by the pectoral branch of the thoracoacromial artery. The sternocostal head arises from the manubrium and sternum, the costal portion of the first 6 ribs, and the aponeurosis of the external oblique muscle. Innervation of the proximal half to two-thirds of the sternocostal head is also by the lateral pectoral nerve, whereas the inferior portion is by the medial pectoral nerve (C8–T1). Blood is supplied primarily by the lateral thoracic artery. The tendinous portions of both heads converge and attach to the lateral lip of the bicipital groove. The primary function of the pectoralis major is to adduct and internally rotate the humerus; it can also extend the arm.

#### Indications
The most common indications for use of the pectoralis for restoration of elbow flexion are brachial plexopathy and arthrogryposis. Historically, it has been used for the treatment of poliomyelitis as well.

#### Contraindications
Complete brachial plexopathy, compromised pectoralis strength (<M4), elbow contracture that has not or cannot be corrected, tissue disequilibrium, cognitive impairment that precludes rehabilitation and meaningful use, and an unmotivated patient are relative contraindications for a pectoralis transfer. Some investigators discourage using the pectoralis major transfer in women secondary to cosmetic concerns.

#### Review of pectoralis transfer options
**Tendon transfer** Release of the insertion of the pectoralis major tendon with transfer to the bicep muscle was described by Schulze-Berge in 1917.[1] This technique also may be referred to as a pectoralis flexorplasty. Over the years, surgeons began to transfer the pectoralis tendon into the biceps tendon with and without interpositional tendon

graft. Tendon transfer to the ulna also has been reported.

**Unipolar transfer** Clark described a unipolar pectoralis major transfer technique, mobilizing the lower 2.5 inches of the sternocostal head from its origin and transferring it to the biceps tendon through a subcutaneous tunnel.[2] This technique has been modified by adding a strip of fascia from the rectus abdominis inferiorly to provide more substantial tissue to transfer into the biceps tendon. Care must be taken to protect the neurovascular pedicle while elevating the pectoralis.

Transfer of the entire origin of the sternocostal and clavicular heads while maintaining its tendinous insertion on the humerus was later described by Seddon.[3]

**Bipolar transfer** Bipolar transfer (**Fig. 1**) of a portion or the entire pectoralis major also has been described.[4] With this operation, both origin and insertion are completely released and the muscle is rotated on its neurovascular pedicle. A new origin and insertion of the muscle is created. Initial descriptions recommended suturing the pectoralis tendon into the coracoid process and mobilizing the sternocostal origin for transfer distally. Carroll and Kleinman's[4] technique recommended transferring the pectoralis major tendon to the acromion while the origins of the clavicular and sternocostal heads with fascia of the rectus abdominis were tubularized and transferred into the biceps tendon distally. The investigators indicated that their modification placed the transfer into a position that was in alignment with the native position of the biceps and increased the mechanical advantage compared with other previously described techniques. Other investigators have transferred the pectoralis minor along with the major in a unipolar fashion.

#### Results
Multiple studies have reported small case series to accompany their surgical technique. Brooks and Seddon[5] reported on 10 patients in whom the pectoralis major tendon was released from the humerus and transferred into the long head of the biceps tendon. Nine of the 10 patients obtained at least M3 or M4 strength. One patient obtained M2 strength and was considered a failure. No patients obtained M5 strength. Active range of motion (AROM) in the successful patients was from 20° to "full" flexion. Beaton and colleagues[6] also evaluated pectoralis flexorplasty with fascia lata as an interposition graft. The mean AROM in their group of 5 patients was 25/116°. The mean strength at 90° of elbow flexion was 16% of the contralateral extremity.

Three of the 4 patients treated with bipolar pectoralis major transfer by Carroll and Kleinman[4] obtained

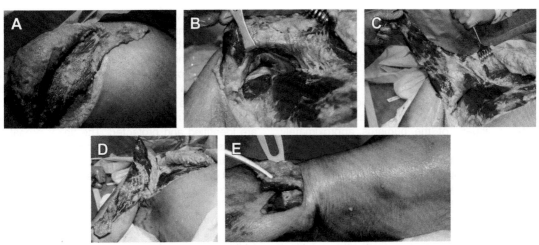

**Fig. 1.** Bipolar pectoralis major transfer. The patient is placed supine and an inframammary incision allows for release of the sternal and costal origins along with an extension of rectus abdominis fascia (*A*). The neurovascular pedicle is exposed to allow for mobilization of the pectoralis major (*B*). The muscle is then rotated on the pedicle (*C*), and the planned transfer is demonstrated (*D*). After securing the proximal aspect of the muscle to the acromion and lateral clavicle, the rectus fascia is passed through a subcutaneous tunnel to allow for transfer to the distal biceps (*E*). Tubularizing this fascia improves the ability to suture this to the distal biceps.

elbow flexion greater than 120°. A series of bipolar transfers in 4 patients by Botte and Wood[7] demonstrated AROM of 25/125° and strength of M3+ to M4. Marshall and colleagues[8] reported on 11 patients who had a pectoralis major to biceps transfer. This series used 2 separate techniques (Clark's procedure or Carroll and Kleinman's[4] procedure) and reported that 9 of the 11 patients failed to obtain 90° of flexion. The average flexion was 34°. The investigators believed the high failure rate was related to poor preoperative strength or shoulder instability.

## Steindler Flexorplasty

### Introduction
Use of the flexor-pronator mass to restore elbow flexion was first documented by Steindler in 1918.[9] Initially this procedure was performed in patients with poliomyelitis; however, it has been expanded to individuals with traumatic or birth brachial plexus palsies, cerebral palsy, and arthrogryposis.

### Anatomy
The flexor-pronator mass is composed of the musculature that originates from the medial epicondyle of the humerus. Included in this group is the pronator teres, palmaris longus, flexor carpi radialis, flexor digitorum superficialis, and the humeral head of the flexor carpi ulnaris (FCU). The latter muscle is innervated by the ulnar nerve (C8 and T1), and the former muscles are innervated by the median nerve (C6–C8). Blood to the flexor-pronator mass is supplied by muscular branches of the radial and ulnar arteries. The primary function of the flexor-pronator mass is to pronate the

forearm, flex the wrist, and flex the digits at the proximal interphalangeal joints, but these muscles are also capable of weak elbow flexion.

### Indications
Current use of the Steindler flexorplasty is commonly limited to patients with brachial plexus palsies involving weakness or complete loss of active elbow flexion. The procedure also can be performed in patients with arthrogryposis. Some surgeons recommend that patients undergoing the procedure must be able to perform a "Steindler effect." This phenomenon is demonstrated by actively pronating the forearm and flexing the wrist while attempting to swing the elbow into flexion. Patients should have strong wrist and digital flexors.

### Contraindications
Contraindications of the Steindler flexorplasty include paralysis or significant weakness of the flexor-pronator mass including wrist flexion. This scenario is particularly seen in extended upper brachial plexus palsies that involve the C5, C6, and C7 nerve roots. High failure rates have been reported when strength is less than M4. Investigators also have recommended that the Steindler flexorplasty should be performed only when there is at least some intact active elbow flexion, as the procedure alone has insufficient strength for useful elbow flexion. Other contraindications include significant unresolved elbow extension or flexion contractures, complete pan-plexus brachial plexus palsy, tissue disequilibrium, and a cognitively impaired or unmotivated patient.

### Surgical technique evolution

Steindler[9] described the procedure of proximal transposition of the flexor-pronator mass to restore elbow flexion almost century ago. The original technique recommended suturing the flexor-pronator mass to the medial intermuscular septum. Mayer and Green[10] modified this technique by moving the fixation site of the flexor-pronator mass to the anterior aspect of the humerus approximately 5 cm proximal to the medial epicondyle. These investigators commented that fixation to the humerus was more robust than the intermuscular septum and the more lateral placement reduced "pronatory" effect of the muscles, thus reducing the propensity for pronation contractures. This modification has become accepted as the standard surgical technique and is known as the modified Steindler flexorplasty.

### Surgical technique

A curvilinear incision centered over the medial epicondyle is extended proximally and distally (**Fig. 2**). Branches of the medial antebrachial cutaneous nerves are protected. The ulnar nerve is identified and an in situ cubital tunnel release is performed, thus allowing the nerve to be protected throughout the case. The fascia between the 2 heads of the FCU is divided for at least 5 cm distal to the medial epicondyle. The distal portion of the medial intermuscular septum is excised. The median nerve and brachial artery are identified and protected. The flexor-pronator mass is then isolated using a hemostat from anteriorly and is placed under the muscle distal to the medial epicondyle and protrudes posteriorly adjacent to the ulnar nerve. The medial epicondyle is predrilled if a screw is to be placed. The medial epicondyle is then osteotomized (adults) or the apophysis is elevated completely using a scalpel (children), thus mobilizing the entire humeral origin of the flexor-pronator mass. Care must be taken to protect the origin of the medial collateral ligament, which is slightly more inferior and lateral. The musculature is then elevated and mobilized distally to allow for proximal and lateral transfer. The biceps muscle, median nerve, and brachial

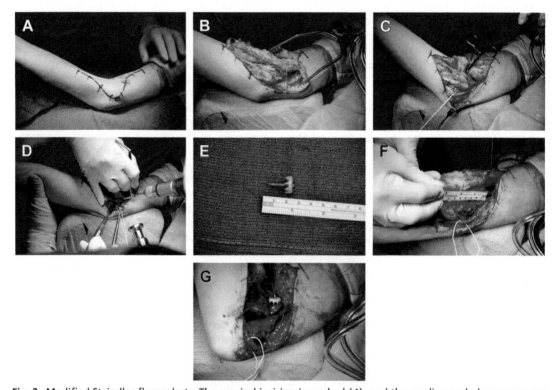

**Fig. 2.** Modified Steindler flexorplasty. The surgical incision is marked (*A*), and the median and ulnar nerves are exposed and protected (*B*). The plane deep to the flexor-pronator mass is developed, and a hemostat is placed in this plane (*C*). The medial epicondyle is predrilled before osteotomy (*D*) to accommodate the 3.5-mm screw with soft tissue washer (*E*). The planned transfer site is measured 5 cm proximal to medial epicondyle in the midportion of the humerus from medial to lateral (*F*). The recipient site is lightly decorticated and drilled, and the transfer is secured a with the 3.5-mm screw over a spiked washer (*G*). Fixation also may be augmented with 1 to 2 suture anchors.

artery are retracted laterally and the brachialis muscle is divided longitudinally. The anterior humerus is exposed approximately 5 cm proximal to the medial epicondyle. Superficial decortication of the humerus is performed and the medial epicondyle is fixed with a 3.5-mm screw and washer with the elbow in approximately 80° of flexion. Several methods of fixation of the flexor-pronator mass also have been described, including wires, suture, suture anchors, and k-wires. Hemostasis is obtained and the wound is closed. The elbow is splinted in approximately 90° of flexion with the forearm in 20 to 30° of supination.

### Results

Several important points should be considered when analyzing the results of the modified Steindler flexorplasty. Moving the point of origin of the flexor-pronator mass proximally by 5 to 7 cm decreases the ability to extend the elbow due to a tethering effect. Because of this, residual elbow flexion contractures are to be expected. Second, the tightening of the flexor-pronator mass by proximal transfer also results in loss of active supination. Patients may also develop a "Steindler effect," which results in forearm pronation and wrist flexion as the elbow is actively flexed. This effect can reduce the patient's ability to supinate the forearm as the hand approaches the mouth.

Recent studies on the modified Steindler procedure have been more in depth in reporting range of motion, strength, and patient-related outcome scales. Ishida and colleagues[11] reported a mean AROM (MAROM) of the elbow of 42 to 107° in 11 patients. Strength was considered grade 4 or 5 in 8 patients and grade 3 in 2 patients. Five patients were able to lift 5 kg. Chen[12] reported a MAROM of 34 to 116° and the ability to lift 3.3 kg. The series of Beaton and colleagues[6] demonstrated a MAROM of 20 to 117°. The mean pronation and supination was 76 and 30° respectively. Liu and colleagues[13] reported MAROM of 28 to 142°, pronation of 74°, and supination of 30°. Seventy-eight percent were able to lift at least 2 kg and the other 22% were able to lift 1 kg. Eggers and colleagues,[14] in a series of 4 patients, reported that 3 patients obtained an 80° arc of flexion (30–115) and 1 patient had a 55° arc of flexion (60–115). The average strength was 0.8 kg (range 0.35–1 kg). Dutton and Dawson[15] reported a mean arc of flexion of 95°, MAROM of 36 to 131°, and mean pronation and supination of 79° and 51°, respectively.

The most common significant complications of the modified Steindler flexorplasty are inadequate elbow flexion and weakness. Patients may not be able to reach their mouth and may not have enough strength for activities that require elbow flexion. The main cause of this complication is inadequate strength of the flexor-pronator mass before the procedure. Careful preoperative strength assessment is paramount to prevent a compromised outcome. Failure of fixation to the anterior humerus also can contribute to a poor result. Finally, care also must be taken when dissecting out the ulnar and median nerves to prevent injury.

### Latissimus Transfer

Latissimus transfer for elbow flexion was first described by Schottstaedt and colleagues[16] and Hovnanian.[17] These investigators described a unipolar technique in which the humeral insertion was not altered, whereas Zancolli and Mitre[18] described a bipolar technique. In the bipolar technique, the origin and insertion sites of the latissimus are released, and the muscle is mobilized on its pedicle to establish a new origin and insertion. Proximal fixation to the coracoid can help to stabilize the shoulder while also creating a direct line of pull to the transferred insertion site at the biceps, radial tuberosity, or proximal ulna.

The latissimus dorsi is a large muscle that originates from the lumbosacral and thoracolumbar portions of the spine and inserts on the humeral shaft. The blood supply is from the thoracodorsal artery, which is a branch of the subscapular artery. The thoracodorsal nerve, derived from the C5, C6, and C7 nerve roots, innervates the muscle. The artery, nerve, and 1 to 2 venae comitantes run for approximately 7 to 10 cm and then penetrate along the anterior aspect of the muscle. This long pedicle allows for extensive mobilization of the muscle. The latissimus function is primarily adduction, internal rotation, and extension of the arm. Donor morbidity is minimal following the procedure due to compensatory function of the teres major.

Assessing the latissimus dorsi as a potential donor for elbow flexion is extremely important, particularly in the case of brachial plexus injury, in which the muscle may be partially or completely denervated. To preoperatively assess latissimus function, arm adduction against resistance while palpating the latissimus can be performed. This is a useful method to assess latissimus function, but it can be difficult to differentiate the latissimus from teres major with this test. The latissimus muscle also can be palpated at the posterior axillary fold as the patient coughs and if noted to contract it may be acceptable for transfer. Another helpful examination technique for preoperative assessment is to lie the patient prone and ask the patient to extend the arm and adduct toward the midline against resistance. The latissimus is visible and palpable with this maneuver.

Grade M4 latissimus strength or greater is required for transfer, and preoperative strength predicts postoperative strength.[19]

### Indications

The most common indications for latissimus transfer to restore elbow flexion are soft tissue injury to the anterior compartment of the arm and upper trunk (C5–6) brachial plexus injuries. An advantage of selecting the latissimus as the donor muscle is that the transfer may be performed as a myocutaneous flap for concomitant soft tissue coverage.

Advantages of bipolar latissimus transfer over unipolar transfer are (1) increased elbow flexion strength, (2) increased shoulder stabilization by fixation to the coracoid process, and (3) improved shoulder flexion.

### Contraindications

A poorly functioning latissimus muscle should not be transferred, as the muscle loses power through the transfer. Limitation in passive elbow range of motion is a relative contraindication. Inexperience with the technique is another relative contraindication, as this is a more technically demanding procedure than the other muscle transfer options for restoration of elbow flexion.

### Surgical technique

The procedure may be performed with the patient in the supine or in the lateral decubitus position. When harvesting the latissimus, the lateral decubitus position affords greater access to the muscle, particularly the midline origin (**Fig. 3**A). Placing the patient in the lateral position initially for the harvest and then rolling the patient supine for the transfer portion of the procedure allows for ideal exposure for both the harvesting and transferring portions of the procedure. A longitudinal incision is made at the anterior edge of the latissimus up to the axilla. The incision includes a cutaneous paddle when needed for soft tissue coverage. The neurovascular pedicle is identified and protected while mobilizing the latissimus muscle. The muscle is completely released from its origin such that the neurovascular pedicle is its sole tether (**Fig. 3**B). Mobilization requires division of the circumflex scapular artery and serratus anterior branches. When performing the bipolar transfer, the latissimus is released off of its humeral insertion. The tendinous portion is then passed under the pectoralis major insertion and is then attached to the coracoid process and conjoined tendon (**Fig. 3**C). A deltopectoral incision may be used as well to accomplish this, but extending the incision into the axilla and retracting the pectoralis major in a cephalad direction will also allow for passage of the tendon and attachment to the coracoid. The surgeon must be very cognizant not to twist the

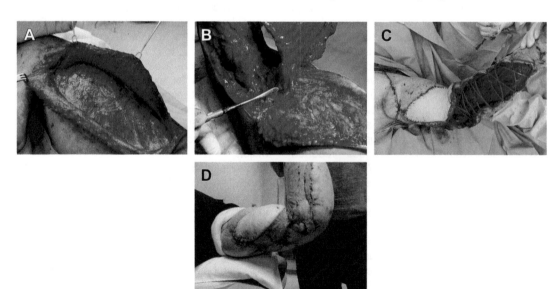

**Fig. 3.** Latissimus dorsi transfer. The patient is placed in the lateral decubitus position to allow for wide exposure of the latissimus dorsi (*A*). The muscle is completely released from its origin and insertion so that it is freely mobilized on its pedicle (*B*). In this case, the patient sustained a severe traumatic injury, with loss of nearly the entire anterior compartment of the arm. A bipolar pedicled latissimus transfer was performed with a large myocutaneous flap that provided soft tissue coverage. In addition, the muscle was transferred to the coracoid and biceps tendon insertion (*C*). Following skin grafting, the wound healed completely (*D*). (*Courtesy of* Ryan Garcia, MD, Charlotte, NC.)

pedicle to avoid ischemia and engorgement of the muscle. If soft tissue injury to the anterior arm is present, the incision is extended down the anterior arm. Otherwise, a large subcutaneous soft tissue tunnel may be created and a separate incision is placed at the elbow flexion crease.

Proximal fixation is accomplished with a combination of heavy, nonabsorbable suture to the conjoined tendon and periosteum of the coracoid. The portion of harvested muscle from the spine and lumbar fascia is tubularized and sutured into the biceps and/or proximal ulna[20] distally. If the biceps tendon is of good quality and remains attached to the radial tuberosity, the muscle is sutured directly to the tendon. Otherwise, the muscle may be fixed directly to the radial tuberosity with a cortical button or transosseous sutures. The muscle also may be split and transferred to the proximal ulna. In this technique, the muscle is passed through a subcutaneous tunnel medially and a dorsal incision is made to allow for transosseous fixation to the ulna.

Soft tissue tensioning is performed such that the elbow rests in approximately 100° of flexion when the distal fixation is performed. A quilting suture technique is used to tack down the dead space of the donor site over multiple drains to reduce the risk of seroma formation. Drains may need to stay in place for 1 to 2 weeks postoperatively.

Postoperatively, the elbow is immobilized in approximately 100° of flexion for 6 weeks. In the case of myocutaneous transfer, viability of the muscle may be monitored by inspection of the transferred cutaneous flap. Active elbow flexion is then encouraged in physical therapy. Gradual, progressive elbow extension is then permitted as the patient demonstrates the ability to actively flex the elbow. Recovery is gradual, and strength may improve for 6 months or more postoperatively (**Fig. 3**D).

### Results

Strength assessment may be performed at 6 months or more postoperatively. Of 71 cases, 76% of patients recovered elbow flexion strength against resistance for cases reported between 1973 and 2008.[20] Flexion power averages 2 to 3 kg.[8,20–22] Mild to moderate improvements in supination of 10 to 50° also have been reported.[18,23,24] Mild flexion contractures of 10 to 15° are common.[18,20]

Patients with functioning forearm and digital flexors appear to achieve greater elbow flexion than patients with paralytic forearm and hand. This is likely a result of the "Steindler effect," in which flexion of the flexor-pronator mass contributes to elbow flexion.

Two studies demonstrated that latissimus transfers for elbow flexion produced superior results as compared to the Steindler flexorplasty.[14,21]

### Triceps to Biceps

Originally described as a transfer of the entire triceps to the biceps by Bunnell in 1951[25] and then Carroll in 1952.[26] This produces a strong transfer, but results in a loss of active elbow extension. A 10-year follow-up review of patients with arthrogryposis who underwent this procedure demonstrated that a disabling elbow flexion contracture resulted in most patients.[27]

Haninec and Szeder[28] described transfer of a pedicled long head of triceps for reconstruction of elbow flexion, and Naidu and colleagues[29] subsequently reported a case report of a patient treated with this procedure. The major advantage of this procedure compared with a complete triceps to biceps transfer is that independent active elbow extension can be maintained. Preoperative electromyography (EMG) of the long head of the triceps demonstrated independent activity separate from the lateral and medial heads.[29]

### Indications

The authors view the complete triceps to biceps transfer as the least favorable option discussed in this article because of the loss of active elbow flexion produced by the procedure. Active elbow extension is necessary for pushing up and out of a chair, for any activities requiring pushing downward, and for use of the hand away from the body for any overhead activities. For these reasons, this transfer is recommended only when other transfers are not available. A rare indication for triceps transfer described by Hoang and colleagues[30] is when simultaneous co-contraction of the triceps and biceps is seen following brachial plexus surgery or spontaneous recovery. If uncoordinated contraction of the biceps and triceps reduces active elbow flexion, the investigators recommended consideration of triceps to biceps transfer. Isolated long head of triceps to biceps transfer has been reported in 2 case reports[28,29] and a case series.[31] In the setting of arthrogryposis, passive flexion of approximately 90° is preferred.

### Contraindications

The presence of lower extremity conditions that require use of upper extremity assistive devices, such as crutches, is a contraindication for the procedure, due to the loss of function that would be sacrificed with a loss of active elbow extension. Poor passive elbow flexion is also a contraindication. Prior triceps lengthening and capsular release is a relative contraindication in the case of arthrogryposis due to the tendon being scarred, but this can be overcome with use of a graft to bypass the scarred tendon.

### Surgical technique

**Triceps to biceps transfer** The patient is placed supine, and a posterior incision is used to reflect the triceps from medial to lateral off of the posterior aspect of the humerus and from its insertion on the olecranon (**Fig. 4**). The ulnar nerve is dissected out as the medial aspect of the triceps is mobilized. The triceps is passed through a lateral subcutaneous tunnel to the anterior aspect of the elbow, and a separate incision is made in the elbow flexion crease to allow for the triceps to biceps transfer. The biceps tendon is exposed and a Pulvertaft weave is then carried out with the elbow in approximately 90° of flexion.

**Isolated long head of triceps to biceps transfer** When considering an isolated long head of triceps transfer, an EMG may be obtained to confirm distinct innervation of the long head from the lateral and medial heads. In the case of arthrogryposis, this is not necessary. The patient is placed supine. With the selective transfer of the long head of the triceps, a medial incision or long straight posterior incision is used to identify the vascular pedicle to the long head of the triceps. Dissection of this pedicle leads to the radial nerve branch to the long head of triceps, which is the first branch of the radial nerve and is found approximately 10 cm distal to the acromion. It is not necessary to dissect out the neurovascular pedicle. Shoulder abduction and elbow flexion put the long head of triceps on maximal stretch, which is then bluntly dissected out from the medial head. The long head tendon insertion, which is the medial one-third to one-half of the entire triceps insertion, is then released sharply off of the olecranon along with an extension of FCU fascia, which is needed for achieving appropriate length.

The target for transfer may be the biceps tendon, radial tuberosity, or proximal ulna. Naidu and colleagues[29] describe palmaris longus harvest for

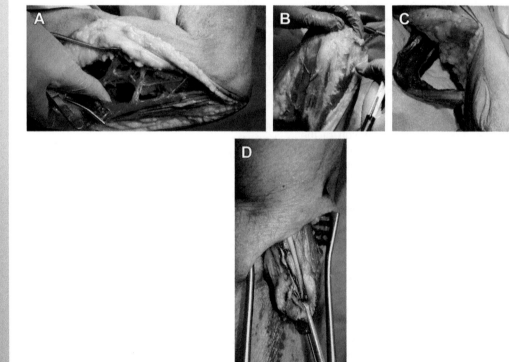

**Fig. 4.** Triceps to biceps transfer. The radial nerve is identified at the lateral border of the triceps, and the triceps is mobilized from the posterior humeral shaft (*A*). The triceps insertion is exposed for planned release (*B*). After mobilizing the medial triceps from the ulnar nerve and releasing it from the olecranon, the triceps is passed through a lateral, subcutaneous tunnel to an incision in the antecubital fossa (*C*). The triceps is passed through the antecubital incision to allow for transfer to the biceps or radial tuberosity (*D*).

attachment to the radial tuberosity, which is accessed through the interval between brachioradialis and pronator teres. The investigators describe that the arm is then extended and the long head of triceps is tensioned to the proximal aspect of the palmaris graft. Gogola and colleagues[31] prefer transfer to the proximal ulna, which is accomplished by the FCU fascia extension of the triceps or with a fascia lata graft.

Postoperatively, with either technique, the patient is placed into a long arm splint at approximately 110° of flexion for 4 weeks and is then transitioned into a hinged elbow brace with progressive elbow extension.

## Results

Hoang and colleagues[30] reported 5 of 7 patients who underwent triceps to biceps transfer were able to get their hand to their mouth. Active elbow flexion arc averaged 123° with a mean loss of 13° of passive elbow extension. These patients were able to support an average of 3.3 kg (range, 1–5 kg) at 90° of elbow flexion. All 7 patients reported significant functional improvement. For

**Table 1**
**Summary and results of muscle transfers to restore elbow flexion**

| Transfer | Advantages | Disadvantages | Results |
|---|---|---|---|
| Pectoralis major: flexorplasty, unipolar or bipolar | Good power | • Poor cosmetic effect.<br>• Can destabilize the shoulder.<br>• May be partially denervated in C5–6 palsy | Flexorplasty: 9/10 M3–4, active range of motion (AROM) 20°–"full" flexion[5]<br>Flexorplasty: mean AROM: 25°–116°, strength 16% of contralateral side[6]<br>Bipolar: 3 of 4 flexion >120°[4]<br>Bipolar: 4/4 M3–4, AROM: 25°–125°[7]<br>Unipolar or bipolar: 2/11 >90° flexion[8] |
| Steindler flexorplasty | Less technically demanding | • Weak power following transfer<br>• Can result in elbow flexion contracture<br>• Requires simultaneous wrist and digital flexion | • 8/11 M4–5,[11] 11/12 M4[32]<br>• Mean elbow flexion strength 0.8–3.3 kg[12–14]<br>• Mean active flexion: 107°–142°[6,11–15]<br>• Mean flexion contracture: 20°–42°[6,11–15] |
| Latissimus dorsi: unipolar or bipolar | • Good power<br>• May be transferred as myocutaneous flap<br>• Minimal donor site morbidity | • Larger surgery<br>• Technically more challenging surgery<br>• May destabilize the shoulder | • 76% M4[14,18–21,23,33]<br>• Mean flexion power 2–3 kg[14,18–21,23,33]<br>• Mean active flexion 91° (45°–130°) |
| Triceps to biceps: total or isolated long head transfer | • Fair power<br>• Less technically demanding procedure<br>• Independent elbow flexion and extension with long head transfer | • Total triceps transfer sacrifices active elbow extension<br>• Severe elbow flexion contractures may develop in long term[27] | Total triceps transfer: 5/7 M4 hand to mouth, active flexion arc 123°, mean 3.3 kg flexion strength[30]<br>Long head triceps transfer: 2/2 M4 elbow flexion with preserved M3 elbow extension[28,29] |

patients with arthrogryposis who underwent this procedure, disabling elbow flexion contractures developed in most patients at 10-year follow-up.[27]

Isolated long head of the triceps to biceps transfer with a palmaris longus graft was reported in 1 patient to achieve active elbow range of motion from 10 to 110° with grade 4 strength.[29] Clinical observation and EMG study demonstrated independent activation of the long head of the triceps with elbow flexion, and activation of the medial and lateral heads occurred with elbow extension.[29]

## SUMMARY

Restoration of elbow flexion after brachial plexus injury, anterior arm trauma, or in the case of arthrogryposis can be accomplished by multiple techniques. Nerve transfers or nerve grafting procedures are often preferred in the early postinjury period, but are less favorable when the target muscle is destroyed or atrophied. Muscle transfers using pectoralis major, the flexor-pronator mass, triceps, or latissimus dorsi are all capable of restoring elbow flexion. The choice of transfer must be individualized based on donor muscle availability and patient preference (**Table 1**). Complete triceps transfer produces the greatest deficit due to sacrifice of active elbow flexion and in the long term results in significant elbow flexion contracture. Isolated long head of triceps transfer is appealing, but clinical evidence is limited. The cosmetic defect produced by pectoralis major transfer must be discussed with patients preoperatively, especially female patients. The Steindler flexorplasty is reliable, but produces weak elbow flexion. Latissimus transfers overall provide the greatest increase in strength with minimal donor site morbidity, and have the added benefit of being transferred as a myocutaneous flap to provide soft tissue coverage to the anterior arm when needed.

## REFERENCES

1. Schulze-Berge VSR. Ersatz der Beuger des Vorderarmes (Bizceps und Brachialis) durch den Pectoralis major. Dtsch Med Wochenschr 1917;43:433.
2. Clark JMP. Reconstruction of the biceps brachii by pectoral muscle transplantation. Br J Surg 1946;34:180.
3. Seddon HJ. Symposium on Reconstructive Surgery of Paralyzed upper limb: Transplantation of pectoralis major for paralysis of the flexors of the elbow. Proc Roy Soc Med 1949;42:837–8.
4. Carroll RE, Kleinman WB. Pectoralis major transplantation to restore elbow flexion to the paralytic limb. J Hand Surg Am 1979;4(6):501–7.
5. Brooks DM, Seddon HJ. Pectoral transplantation for paralysis of the flexors of the elbow. Bone Joint J 1959;41B(1):36–43. Available at: http://www.bjj.boneandjoint.org.uk/content/41-B/1/36.abstract.
6. Beaton DE, Dumont A, Mackay MB, et al. Steindler and pectoralis major flexorplasty: a comparative analysis. J Hand Surg Am 1995;20(5):747–56.
7. Botte MJ, Wood MB. Flexorplasty of the elbow. Clin Orthop Relat Res 1989;245:110–6.
8. Marshall RW, Williams DH, Birch R, et al. Operations to restore elbow flexion after brachial plexus injuries. J Bone Joint Surg Br 1988;70(4):577–82.
9. Steindler A. Operative treatment of paralytic conditions of the upper extremity. J Orthop Surg 1919;1:608–19.
10. Mayer L, Green W. Experiences with the Steindler flexorplasty at the elbow. J Bone Joint Surg Am 1954;36(4):775–862. Available at: http://jbjs.org/content/36/4/775.abstract.
11. Ishida O, Sunagawa T, Suzuki OO, et al. Modified Steindler procedure for the treatment of brachial plexus injuries. Arch Orthop Trauma Surg 2006;126(1):63–5.
12. Chen WS. Restoration of elbow flexion by modified Steindler flexorplasty. Int Orthop 2000;24(1):43–6.
13. Liu TK, Yang RS, Sun JS. Long-term results of the Steindler flexorplasty. Clin Orthop Relat Res 1993;296:104–8.
14. Eggers IM, Mennen U, Matime AM. Elbow flexorplasty: a comparison between latissimus dorsi transfer and Steindler flexorplasty. J Hand Surg Am 1992;17(5):522–5.
15. Dutton RO, Dawson EG. Elbow flexorplasty: an analysis of long-term results. J Bone Joint Surg Am 1981;63(7):1064–9.
16. Schottstaedt ER, Larsen LJ, Bost FC. Complete muscle transposition. Journal of Bone & Joint Surgery American Volume 1955;37-A:897–919.
17. Hovnanian AP. Latissimus dorsi transplantation for loss of flexion or extension at the elbow; a preliminary report on technic. Ann Surg 1956;143(4):493–9. Available at: http://www.ncbi.nlm.nih.gov/pubmed/13303086. Accessed March 5, 2016.
18. Zancolli E, Mitre H. Latissimus dorsi transfer to restore elbow flexion. An appraisal of eight cases. J Bone Joint Surg Am 1973;55(6):1265–75. Available at: http://www.ncbi.nlm.nih.gov/pubmed/4758039. Accessed March 5, 2016.
19. Kawamura K, Yajima H, Tomita Y, et al. Restoration of elbow function with pedicled latissimus dorsi myocutaneous flap transfer. J Shoulder Elbow Surg 2007;16(1):84–90.
20. Cambon-Binder A, Belkheyar Z, Durand S, et al. Elbow flexion restoration using pedicled latissimus dorsi transfer in seven cases. Chir Main 2012;31(6):324–30.
21. Chuang DCC, Epstein MD, Yeh MC, et al. Functional restoration of elbow flexion in brachial plexus

injuries: results in 167 patients (excluding obstetric brachial plexus injury). J Hand Surg Am 1993;18(2): 285–91.

22. Takami H, Takahashi S, Ando M. Latissimus dorsi transplantation to restore elbow flexion to the paralysed limb. J Hand Surg Am 1984;9(1):61–3.

23. Stern PJ, Carey JP. The latissimus dorsi flap for reconstruction of the brachium and shoulder. J Bone Joint Surg Am 1988;70(4):526–35.

24. Nagano A, Ochiai N, Okinaga S. Restoration of elbow flexion in root lesions of brachial plexus injuries. J Hand Surg Am 1992;17(5):815–21. Available at: http://www.ncbi.nlm.nih.gov/pubmed/1401788. Accessed March 6, 2016.

25. Bunnell S. Restoring flexion to the paralytic elbow. J Bone Joint Surg Am 1951;33(3):566–90. Available at: http://jbjs.org/content/33/3/566.abstract.

26. Carroll RE. Restoration of flexor power to the flail elbow by transplantation of the triceps tendon. Surg Gynecol Obstet 1952;95:685–8.

27. Williams PF. Management of upper limb problems in arthrogryposis. Clin Orthop Relat Res 1985;194:60–7.

28. Haninec P, Szeder V. Reconstruction of elbow flexion by transposition of pedicled long head of triceps brachii muscle. Acta Chir Plast 1999;41(3):82–6. Available at: http://www.ncbi.nlm.nih.gov/pubmed/10641328. Accessed March 5, 2016..

29. Naidu S, Lim A, Looi FAMS, et al. Long head of the triceps transfer for elbow flexion. Plast Reconstr Surg 2007;119(3):45e–7e.

30. Hoang PH, Mills C, Burke FD. Triceps to biceps transfer for established brachial plexus palsy. J Bone Joint Surg Br 1989;71(2):268–71.

31. Gogola GR, Ezaki M, Oishi SN, et al. Long head of the triceps muscle transfer for active elbow flexion in arthrogryposis. Tech Hand Up Extrem Surg 2010;14(2):121–4.

32. Monreal R. Steindler flexorplasty to restore elbow flexion in C5-C6-C7 brachial plexus palsy type. J Brachial Plex Peripher Nerve Inj 2007;2:15.

33. Vekris MD, Beris AE, Lykissas MG, et al. Restoration of elbow function in severe brachial plexus paralysis via muscle transfers. Injury 2008;39:S15–22.

# Radial Nerve Tendon Transfers

Andre Eu-Jin Cheah, MD, MBA[a,b], Jennifer Etcheson, MS[a], Jeffrey Yao, MD[a,*]

## KEYWORDS

- Radial nerve palsy • Tendon transfer • Surgical technique

## KEY POINTS

- The functional deficit seen in radial nerve palsy is the loss of wrist extension with subsequent weak grip, and loss of thumb and finger extension.
- Established radial nerve tendon transfers are divided into 5 groups largely based on the donor for the extensor digitorum communis.
- The appropriate choice of transfer for an individual patient is based on the wrist motion, presence of the palmaris longus, and need for flexor carpi ulnaris function and independent thumb extension/ abduction.
- Surgical technique involves the preparation, routing, and coaptation of the donor and recipient tendons as well as the crucial step of tensioning.
- Good outcomes have been reported for all combinations of tendon transfers. Complications include loss of wrist flexion, inappropriate tensioning, and need for tenolysis.

## INTRODUCTION
### Nature of the Problem

Radial nerve palsy may result from nerve damage secondary to trauma or in the event of surgical resection (eg, in tumor extirpation). For neural injury above the origin of the posterior interosseous nerve (PIN), all active extension will be lost at the wrist joint and metacarpophalangeal joint (MCPJ) of the fingers and thumb (**Table 1**). This loss corresponds to the paralysis of the extensor carpi radialis longus and brevis (ECRL and ECRB) as well as extensor carpi ulnaris (ECU) for the wrist. The extensor digitorum communis (EDC), extensor indicis propius (EIP), and extensor digitorum quinti minimi (EDQM) for the fingers and extensor pollicis longus (EPL) for the thumb are also denervated. In addition, thumb extension and radial abduction will be lost with paralysis of the abductor pollicis longus (APL) and extensor pollicis brevis (EPB). In the case of injury after the PIN branches from the radial nerve proper, wrist extension may be spared, albeit with radial deviation owing to the preservation of isolated ECRL function. Sensory loss when the injury is at the radial nerve proper, before it branches to the PIN and superficial radial sensory nerve (SRN), is confined to the skin over the anatomical snuffbox and rarely disturbs the patient unless a neuroma forms.[1] Often substantial overlap exists between the superficial radial nerve and lateral antebrachial cutaneous nerve distributions. An injury before the radial nerve branches to the PIN and SRN is termed a high radial nerve palsy, whereas an injury to the PIN is termed PIN palsy or a low radial nerve palsy.

Disclosures: The authors have nothing to disclose.
[a] Department of Orthopaedic Surgery, Robert A. Chase Hand & Upper Limb Center, Stanford University Medical Center, 450 Broadway Street, Redwood City, CA 94063, USA; [b] Department of Hand & Reconstructive Microsurgery, National University Hospital, National University Health System, 1E Kent Ridge Road, NUHS Tower Block, Level 11, Singapore 119228, Singapore
* Corresponding author. Department of Orthopaedic Surgery, Robert A. Chase Hand & Upper Limb Center, Stanford University Medical Center, 450 Broadway Street (Mailcode: 6342), Redwood City, CA 94063.
E-mail address: jyao@stanford.edu

Hand Clin 32 (2016) 323–338
http://dx.doi.org/10.1016/j.hcl.2016.03.003
0749-0712/16/$ – see front matter © 2016 Elsevier Inc. All rights reserved.

**Table 1**
**Functional loss in radial nerve palsy with corresponding muscles and portion of the radial nerve affected**

| Function Lost | Muscles Affected | Innervation |
|---|---|---|
| Wrist extension | ECRL | Radial nerve |
| | ECRB | PIN |
| | ECU | |
| Finger extension | EDC | |
| | EDQM | |
| | EIP | |
| Thumb extension | EPL | |
| Thumb abduction | EPB | |
| | APL | |

### Effect on prehension

Prehension has been defined as "all the functions that are put into play when an object is grasped by the hands—intent, permanent sensory control, and a mechanism of grip."[2] The phases of prehension have been described to include the approach, the grip, and the release of grip[3] with radial nerve dysfunction being detrimental to the latter two phases. When these patients are unable to stabilize their wrists, grip strength is attenuated because a decrease of wrist extension power of one grade results in decrease of grip strength by 25% to 50%.[4] The release of grip is adversely affected because finger and thumb extension is required to release an object from grip, although it should be remembered that interphalangeal joint extension is still possible through the action of the intrinsic muscles of the hand.

### Relevant anatomy and patient assessment

In the arm, the radial nerve is the continuation of the posterior cord of the brachial plexus (**Fig. 1**), running posterior to the humerus and from medial to lateral across the spiral groove of the humerus. It then travels in a distal-lateral direction just distal to the spiral groove.[5] It pierces the lateral intermuscular septum at approximately 10 cm proximal to the lateral epicondyle, gives off branches to the brachioradialis (BR) and ECRL, and then divides into the PIN and SRN at the level of the supinator muscle. The PIN travels between the 2 heads of the supinator, which can be a source of compression. The PIN then travels distally in the forearm on the extensor surface of the interosseous membrane to supply the ECRB, ECU, and all the finger and thumb extensors before terminating as a sensory branch to the dorsal wrist capsule. The SRN courses distally under the BR, becomes

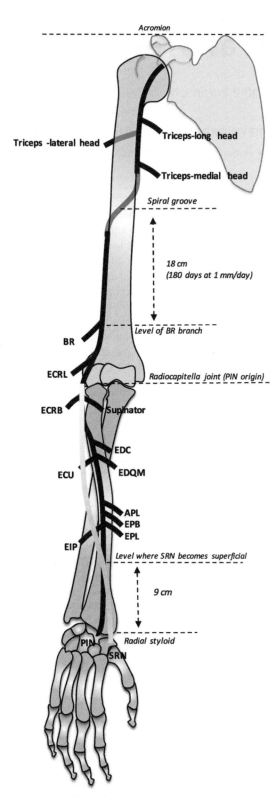

**Fig. 1.** Branches of the radial nerve with relation to bony landmarks; useful when assessing a patient with radial nerve palsy.

subcutaneous approximately 9 cm proximal to the radial styloid, and supplies cutaneous sensation to the anatomical snuffbox, the first web space, and dorsal thumb and index and long fingers. Following an injury to the SRN, a Tinel sign should be elicited along the course of the nerve to help localize the point of injury.

When evaluating a patient with a radial nerve palsy, the time from injury and signs of recovery are important aspects to note in the examination because these factors help determine the need for and the optimal timing of tendon transfer surgery. As a guide, plans should be made for tendon transfer reconstruction if a radial nerve injury at the midshaft humerus does not see return of BR or wrist extension function by 6 months.[6] However, there are investigators who suggest that early tendon transfers may be carried out especially for wrist extension. Early transfers for wrist extension allow an "internal splint" to restore function earlier and at the same time allow for nerve recovery.[4,7] The presence of polyphasics on electromyography may also be useful in determining the potential for spontaneous recovery of function. The examination of the patient with a radial nerve palsy should focus on the functional deficit that needs to be reconstructed as well as the integrity of the potential donors for tendon transfer. Although it is beyond the scope of this article to describe how individual donor and recipient muscles may be assessed, **Table 2** illustrates which muscles the surgeon should focus on. Finally, 2

of the prerequisites for tendon transfer surgery,[8] namely presence of supple joints and soft tissue equilibrium, must be confirmed before any tendon transfers are planned.

In essence, when examining a patient with radial nerve palsy:

1. Attempt to identify the location of the radial nerve injury using Tinel sign along its course.
2. Note the time from injury and assess if recovery is progressing as expected.
3. Assess the functional deficit and integrity of potential donors.
4. Confirm supple joints and soft tissue equilibrium before planning surgery.

## SURGICAL TECHNIQUE
### Preoperative Planning

During the preoperative planning phase for radial nerve tendon transfers, the surgeon should ensure the following:

1. The hand and wrist joints are supple and have full passive range of motion, because postoperative immobilization would accentuate any preexisting stiffness.
2. Definitive skeletal stabilization and soft tissue equilibrium has been achieved.
3. The donor muscle proposed must
   a. Be expendable.
   b. Have adequate strength and excursion[9–11] (see **Table 2**).

**Table 2**
**Excursion (in mm) and relative strength of the usual donor and recipient tendons in radial nerve tendon transfers**

| Role | Function | Muscles | Excursion | Relative Strength |
|------|----------|---------|-----------|-------------------|
| Recipient | Wrist extension | ECRL ECRB ECU | 33 | 1 |
| | Finger extension | EDC EDQM EIP | 50 | 0.5 |
| | Thumb extension | EPL | | 0.1 |
| | Thumb abduction | EPB APL | | |
| Donor | Wrist flexion | PL FCR FCU | 33 | 0.1 1 2 |
| | Forearm pronation | PT | 50 | |
| | Finger flexion | FDS | 70 | 1 |

One of the aims in tendon transfers is to match donor excursion and relative strength to that of the recipient. For example, the PL and its usual recipient the EPL have the same relative strength, whereas the PL has a slightly lower excursion, which can be compensated for by wrist flexion and the tenodesis effect.

c. Have synergistic function with respect to the recipient tendon's function.
d. Have a straight line of pull after weaving to the recipient tendon.
e. Be intended to reconstruct only one function.

Apart from adherence to the general principles of tendon transfers outlined, the authors deem that 4 questions important to radial nerve tendon transfers (specifically restoring finger extension) will help the surgeon tailor the choice of tendon transfers to best suit the patient.

### How good is the patient's wrist motion?

Wrist motion, especially flexion, is important for radial nerve tendon transfers because the tenodesis effect may increase tendon excursion by approximately 30 mm.[12] As a consequence, wrist arthrodesis should be avoided for these patients and preoperative passive range of motion should be maximized through hand therapy efforts. If lack of wrist motion is still a concern, consideration should be made to use the flexor digitorum superficialis (FDS) as a donor to the EDC owing to its increased excursion when compared with the wrist flexors[8] (see **Table 2**).

### How important is flexor carpi ulnaris function to the patient?

The "dart-throwing motion" (DTM) is the one of the most regularly used planes of wrist motion in both occupational and recreational activities that brings the wrist from radial extension to ulnar flexion.[13] The DTM involves mainly the action of the ECRL and flexor carpi ulnaris (FCU),[14] and as such, consideration for reconstruction (or preservation) of the function of these muscles is important especially in patients whose occupations demand this action (eg, manual laborers).[1] PIN palsy is another situation where preservation of FCU function is important to counteract the action of the intact ECRL to minimize radial deviation of the wrist.[8,15] That being said, many investigators use the FCU as a donor (**Table 3**), and some have reported minimal problems with function or coronal alignment of the wrist.[16,17]

### Does the patient have a palmaris longus?

The absence of the palmaris longus (PL) (**Fig. 2**) varies widely between ethnic groups with absence seen in approximately 20% of Caucasian populations but in only 5% of Asian populations.[18] As the PL is an integral donor for thumb extension or abduction in many combinations of tendon transfers,[19–22] absence of the PL would preclude their use. In such a case, the surgeon should contemplate using the FDS-type tendon

transfers,[10] the split flexor carpi radialis (FCR) transfer[23] (**Fig. 3**), or a transfer that uses the FCU as the sole donor.[24] In the case when the PL is used to attain thumb abduction, consider replacing the PL donor with an FDS, typically of the ring finger.[5,16,20]

### How important is independent thumb extension or abduction to the patient?

Most tendon transfer combinations afford an element of thumb independence either by powering the EPL separately from the EDC[7,10,19,21,25–32] or by the addition of a transfer to the first extensor compartment tendons, namely the APL and/or the EPB.[16,20,22,33] The independence of thumb extension may be useful in some musicians, whereas thumb abduction may be particularly important to people who perform most of their work with a computer keyboard. As such, consideration must given to avoid tendon transfer combinations that use only the FCR or FCU as a single donor for the wrist, fingers, and thumb, attenuating the ability for independent thumb extension and/or abduction.[24,34]

### Making the choice of tendon transfers

Innumerous tendon transfers have been described to treat radial nerve palsy, and all have their advocates who have shown commendable results. The authors have classified some of them based on the donor to the EDC (see **Table 3**):

1. FCU type[21,26–28,35]
2. FCR type[7,19,23,31,32,34]
3. FDS type[10,29,30]
4. FCU or FCR type with thumb abduction reconstruction[16,20,22,33]
5. FCU type without dedicated wrist extension reconstruction[24,33,36]

They also present an algorithm to help guide the choice of tendon transfers to perform (**Fig. 4**), and most importantly, they recommend having a meaningful conversation with the patient to understand their needs and then use the procedure the surgeon is most comfortable with to meet those needs.

### Surgical Approach

The universal principles of safe and adequate surgical access to the structures that need to be operated on apply to these tendon transfers: usually 3 donor tendons from the flexor side and the recipient tendons on the dorsum. These principles translate to at least one incision for the transfers using the FCR as a donor for the EDC,[6,37] 2 for those using the FCU,[27] and 3 when the FDS is used.[10,29,30] If rerouting of the EPL through the first

**Table 3**
The various types of tendon transfers based on the muscle used as the extensor digitorum communis donor and whether dedicated thumb abduction and wrist extension reconstruction have been carried out

| Type | Author, y | Recipient Tendon | | | | | | |
| | | Wrist Extension | | Finger Extension | | Thumb Extension | Thumb Abduction | |
| | | ECRB | ECRL | EDC | EIP | EPL | EPB | APL |
|---|---|---|---|---|---|---|---|---|
| FCU | Jones,[25] 1916 | PT | PT | FCU (III–V) | FCR | FCR | Nil | Nil |
| | Zachary,[28] 1946 | PT | PT | FCU | Nil | PL/BR/FCU | Nil | Nil |
| | Said,[26] 1974 | PT | PT (ECU included) | FCU | FCU | PL/FCR | Nil | Nil |
| | Riordan,[21] 1983 | PT | Nil | FCU | Nil | PL | Nil | Nil |
| | Tubiana,[27] 2002 | PT | PT (ECRL centralized) | FCU | FCU | PL | Nil | Nil |
| FCR | Starr,[31] 1922 | PT | PT | FCR | FCR | PL | PL | PL |
| | Brand,[19] 1975 | PT | Nil | FCR | Nil | PL | Nil | Nil |
| | Tsuge,[7] 1980 | PT | PT[a] | FCR (IM)/FCU[a] | Nil | PL | Nil | Tenodesis |
| | Ishida & Ikuta,[32] 2003 | PT | Nil | FCR (IM) | Nil | PL | Nil | Tenodesis |
| | Lim et al,[23] 2004 | PT | Nil | Split FCR | Nil | Split FCR | Nil | Nil |
| | Al-Qattan,[34] 2012 | PT | Nil | FCR | FCR | FCR | FCR | FCR |
| FDS | Boyes,[10] 1962 | PT | PT | FDSIII (III–V) | FDSIV | FDSIV | FCR | FCR |
| | Chuinard et al,[29] 1978 | PT | PT | FDSIII (III–V) | FDSIV | FDSIV | FCR | FCR |
| | Krishnan & Schackert,[30] 2008 | PT | PT | FDSIV | FDSIII (III–V) | FDSIII (III–V) | Nil | PL |
| FCU/FCR with abduction reconstruction | Merle D'Aubigne,[20] 1949 | PT | PT | FCU | Nil | FCU | PL/FDS | PL/FDS |
| | Brooks,[22] 1984 | PT | Nil | FCU/FCR | Nil | FCU/FCR | PL | Nil |
| | Kruft et al,[33] 1997 | PT | PT | FCU | Nil | FCU | PL | PL |
| | Dunnet et al,[16] 1995 | PT | Nil | FCU/FCR | Nil | FCU/FCR | PL/FDS | Nil |
| FCU without wrist reconstruction | Kruft et al,[33] 1997 | Nil | Nil | FCU (II–V + EDM) | FCU | FCU | Nil | Nil |
| | Gousheh & Arasteh,[24] 2006 | Nil | Nil | FCU | FCU | FCU | Nil | Nil |
| | Monacelli et al,[36] 2011 | Nil | Nil | FCU | FCU | PL | Nil | Nil |

*Abbreviation:* IM, routed through the interosseous membrane.
[a] Previously, but no longer used to perform these transfers.

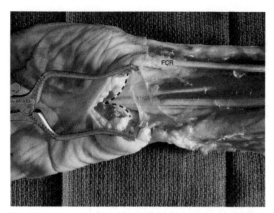

Fig. 2. Volar aspect of a cadaveric left wrist with a missing PL. The proximal transverse carpal ligament (*dotted line*) is divided to expose the finger flexors.

extensor compartment is done, an additional incision at the dorsum of the thumb MCPJ is usually needed.[7,38] In addition, the skin incisions need to be planned such that the tendon weaves do not lie directly under the incisions[1,39] and that the incisions are wide enough to ensure adequate proximal mobilization of the donors such as the pronator teres (PT) and PL.[16] In **Figs. 5** and **6**, an example of a 2-incision design for a FCR-type transfer is shown.

## SURGICAL PROCEDURE
### Step One: Dissection of the Donor Tendons

After making the appropriate surgical incisions for the donors in the tendon transfer combination planned, priority should be given to identifying and protecting cutaneous nerves, such as the SRN (**Fig. 7**), the dorsal sensory branch of the ulnar nerve (DBUN) (**Fig. 8**), and the palmar cutaneous branch of the median nerve (PCB). Similarly, the

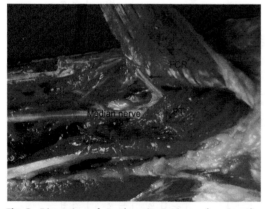

Fig. 3. Dissection of a cadaveric specimen showing the 2 branches of the FCR (*arrows*) that have to be identified if a split FCR transfer is planned. Note that the branches are very proximal and close to each other.

radial and ulnar artery must be identified and protected during the harvest of the FCR and FCU tendons, respectively. The donor muscle bellies must be well mobilized while taking care not to damage their neurovascular pedicles, especially if a split FCR transfer is planned (see **Fig. 3**).[23] In the case of the FCU, which has a muscle belly that extends very distally, an effort should be made to strip the distal tendon end of muscle (**Fig. 9**).[27] If the PT is used for wrist extension, it is important to harvest a distal periosteal strip of tissue to allow sufficient length for tendon transfer.

### Step Two: Preparation of the Recipient Tendons

After surgical access has been gained to the recipient extensor tendons, every effort should be made to clear the fascia surrounding the tendons of extensor compartments one, two, and four *proximally* while preserving the integrity of the extensor retinaculum. This maneuver ensures good gliding of the tendon transfers while minimizing bowstringing if the retinaculum were to be released. Next, the EPL should be identified and removed from the third extensor compartment and incised at its musculotendinous junction to prepare for an end-to-end transfer. The preparation for the ECRB and EDC differs between investigators with some incising these tendons at their musculotendinous junctions to prepare for end-to-end transfer to achieve a straight line of pull,[8,27] while others perform end-to-side transfers.[4,21,29] The latter is usually done when early tendon transfers are performed with the hope of some recovery of radial nerve function, and as a consequence, ECRB and EDC function.

### Step Three: Routing the Donor Tendons to the Recipient Tendons

#### Ensure that the transfers are not compressing the cutaneous nerves
This step involves creating the path for the donor to reach the recipient. When using the subcutaneous route, care must be taken to protect the SRN (see **Fig. 7**), DBUN (see **Fig. 8**), and PCB. When the PT, FCR, or FCU is used as a donor, it good to note that the SRN and DBUN are usually found distal to and away from where these transfers are typically located (**Fig. 10**). When the PL is transferred for thumb animation, however, a subcutaneous tunnel deep to the cutaneous nerves is created and maintained with the help of a vessel loop (**Fig. 11**). When a tunnel through the interosseous membrane is used, the anterior and PIN and artery must be protected, and adequate resection of the IOM must be performed.[29]

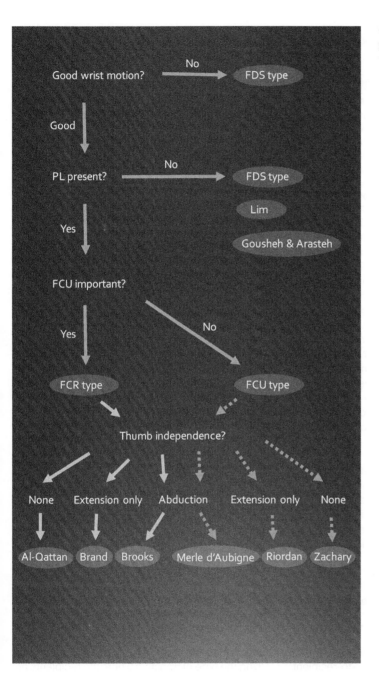

**Fig. 4.** Suggested algorithm for the choice of tendon transfer to offer an individual patient.

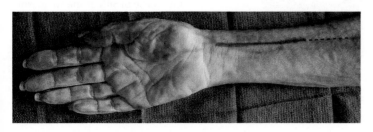

**Fig. 5.** Extensile volar incision along the FCR to gain access to the PT, FCR, and PL if a FCR-type transfer is planned. The dotted line represents the direction that the wound may be extended.

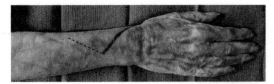

**Fig. 6.** Oblique incision over the extensor surface to gain exposure to the recipient tendons. The incision may be extended proximally (*dotted line*) if better access is needed *proximal* to the extensor retinaculum.

### Paths that the donor tendons may take

For the PT, it is typically routed around the subcutaneous border of the radius,[1,8,37] although some have described routing the PT under the BR instead.[30] For the FCU-type[21,27] and FCR-type[19] transfers, the usual route to the EDC is around the subcutaneous border of the ulna and radius, respectively. For FDS transfers[10,29,30] and certain types of FCR transfers,[7,32] the donor motor is routed to the EDC via two 1 cm × 2 cm openings on either side of the interosseous neurovascular structures proximal to the pronator quadratus.[29] An option to minimize adhesions in this window is to make it larger and detach some of the origin of the FDS muscle belly from the interosseous membrane.[7] Last, the EPL is typically rerouted subcutaneously toward the usual donor (PL) after it is removed from the third extensor compartment to prevent adduction of the thumb when the PL contracts.[19,21] Again, caution must be used to ensure that the EPL-PL transfer passes deep to the SRN and PCB. Occasionally, the EPL may be rerouted retrograde through the first extensor compartment after it is removed at the thumb MCPJ dorsum via a small skin incision to provide thumb abduction.[38] A slip of the APL may be excised to accommodate the EPL.

### Step Four: Weaving the Donor Tendon to the Recipient Tendon

#### Location of weaves

The authors emphasize again that for wrist extension and finger MCPJ, the donor-to-recipient weave should be located proximal to the extensor retinaculum to prevent bowstringing. In addition, these should be proximal enough such that the transfer weaves will not get caught under the extensor retinaculum in wrist and finger MCPJ flexion.

#### Type of weaves

The Pulvertaft weave is the most common method used to connect the donor to the recipient tendon, although there are other methods that have been described (**Fig. 12**).[40] The Pulvertaft weave involves threading the donor tendon through the recipient tendon using multiple (usually 3) orthogonal tunnels, which are secured by horizontal mattress sutures at each of the intersection points. Further refinement for the FCU to EDC transfer has been made by splitting the FCU tendon and only threading one limb through the EDC while using the other limb to refine the tension and reinforce the weave.[21,27]

### Step Five: Tensioning the Transfer

#### The Blix curve and optimal muscle tension

Although dogma advises to set the tension of the donor muscle for the tendon transfer on the high side at approximately 75% of maximal excursion,[12] consideration should be given to setting the transfer when the muscle is at optimal tension and not maximal tension.[40] The Blix curve (**Fig. 13**) informs about optimal sarcomere length, which allows the muscle to generate the maximal contractile force. If the donor muscle is overstretched from a tendon transfer that is tensioned too much, the sarcomere would be set at a length that falls in the passive part of the Blix curve, reducing its contractile force.[41] As such, attention should be paid to setting the muscle close to its natural resting length. Setting the muscle close to its natural resting length may be aided intraoperatively by marking the donor muscle with sutures at fixed intervals before the detachment of its tendon and ensuring that these fixed intervals are maintained after the tendon weave is performed.

#### Order of tensioning

Using the type of transfers where the recipients are the ECRB, EDC, and EPL as an example, the sequence in which the tension of the transfers

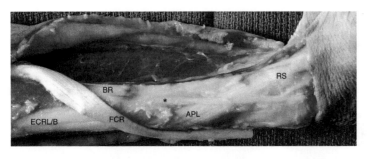

**Fig. 7.** Cadaveric dissection showing the course of SRN at the wrist. Note that the FCR transfer lies *proximal* to the point the SRN (*asterisk*) emerges from under the BR (approximately 9 cm proximal to the radial styloid). The PT and PL transfer will be proximal and distal, respectively, to the FCR transfer.

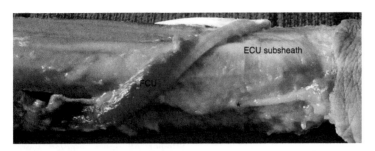

Fig. 8. Cadaveric dissection showing the DBUN (*asterisk*) and the FCU transfer *proximal* to it.

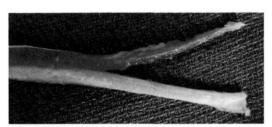

Fig. 9. Note that the muscle belly of the FCU extends very distal and may be trimmed to decrease the bulk of the tendon weave.

may be set are discussed. In general, appropriate tension would require that all 4 fingers extend synchronously and adequately when the wrist is flexed, while all fingers and thumb can be passively flexed into a fist with the wrist extended.

**Wrist transfer first** For investigators that advocate setting the wrist transfer first,[1,42] the PT, at its normal resting length, is woven into the ECRB with the wrist in slight extension (30°–45°). The wrist is then brought to neutral and the FCU or FCR (at its normal resting length) is woven into the EDC with the MCPJ of the fingers in full extension. Last, with the EPL under full tension (and

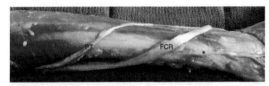

Fig. 10. Cadaveric dissection to show that the SRN (*asterisk*) exits distal to where the PT and FCR transfers are typically found.

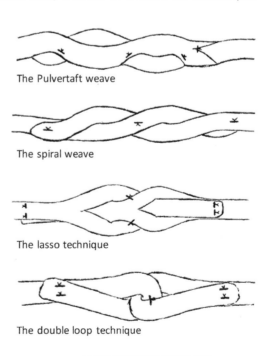

The Pulvertaft weave

The spiral weave

The lasso technique

The double loop technique

The side-to-side technique

Fig. 12. The different types of weaves to coapt the tendons.

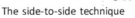

Fig. 11. Intraoperative picture showing the subcutaneous tunnel (held patent by the superior vessel loop) to allow passage of the donor flexor tendons to the recipient extensors *deep* to the SRN. The inferior vessel loop is around a subcutaneous vein.

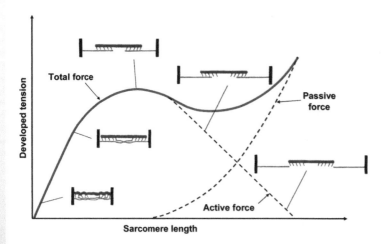

**Fig. 13.** The Blix curve. Note that there is an optimum sarcomere length needed to achieve the peak active force. (*From* Odegard GM, Haut Donahue TL, Morrow DA, et al. Constitutive modeling of skeletal muscle tissue with an explicit strain-energy function. J Biomech Eng 2008;130(6):061017. Copyright © 2016. Used with permission of Elsevier. All rights reserved. www.netterimages.com.)

consequently the thumb MCPJ and interphalangeal joint are in full extension), the PL (at its normal resting length) is woven into the EPL with the wrist in neutral position.

**Wrist transfer last** For those that perform the wrist transfer last, the donors to the EDC and EPL are woven (at their resting length) into these tendons with the wrist in neutral[6] or 45° extension,[27] and the fingers and thumb in full extension. Tension is adjusted until 30° of wrist flexion results in adequate extension of the thumb and finger MCPJs, and wrist extension permits full passive finger flexion. Adequate extension of the fingers refers to restoration of the normal finger cascade where the MCPJs of the fingers are progressively less extended as one moves from radial to ulnar (**Fig. 14**) and is achieved by individually tensioning each EDC to the donor tendon.[27] Last, the PT is woven into the ECRB until a 30° resting posture of the wrist is attained with the MCPJ of the fingers slightly flexed.

### Immediate Postoperative Care

After the skin is closed, the wrist and finger MCPJs are usually immobilized in extension and some flexion, respectively, while the thumb is always in full abduction for 3.5 to 5 weeks (**Table 4**).[1,6,8,16,27,33,37,42,43] The wrist is usually placed in 30° to 50° of extension and the finger MCPJ in 0° to 45° of flexion. Some investigators also advocate placing the forearm in pronation and the elbow in 90° of flexion, to take the tension off the PT transfer while others free the interphalangeal joints of the fingers to minimize stiffness.

### Rehabilitation and Recovery

#### Rehabilitation program

The postprocedure rehabilitation program involves a graduated increase in joint motion, muscle action, and splint weaning (**Table 5**). It must be emphasized that when joint mobilization is commenced at 4 weeks, tension must still be kept off the transfer[8]; this means that elbow flexion and extension must be performed only when the wrist is pronated and extended and when the

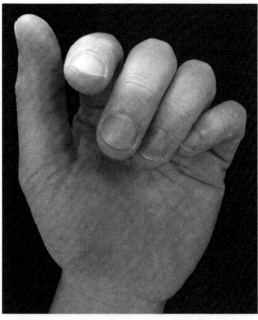

**Fig. 14.** The normal cascade of the fingers. Note that the radial MCPJs are more extended than the ulnar ones.

**Table 4**
The various positions and periods of immobilization used by different investigators

| Author, y | Immobilization (wk) | Elbow Flexion | Forearm Pronation | Wrist Extension | Finger MCPJ Flexion | IPJ Flexion | Thumb MCPJ Flexion | Abduction |
|---|---|---|---|---|---|---|---|---|
| Dunnet et al,[16] 1995 | 3 | Free | NM | 40° | <20° | <20° | NM | NM |
| Kruft et al,[33] 1997 | 3 | NM | NM | 40° | 0° | 0° | 0° | Full |
| Tubiana,[27] 2002 | 3 | NM | 90° | 50° | 15° | Free after 2 wk | 0° | Full |
| Kozin,[43] 2005 | 4–5 | 90° | NM | 45° | 30°–45° | 0° | 0° | Full |
| Sammer & Chung,[8] 2009 | 4 | 90° | 90° | 30° | 0° | Free | 0° | Full |
| Chandraprakasam et al,[37] 2009 | 4 | NM | NM | 30°–40° | 20°–30° | NM | NM | Full |
| Ratner et al,[6] 2010 | NM | NM | NM | 30° | 0° | NM | 0° | Full |
| Jones & Machado,[1] 2011 | 3.5–4 | NM | NM | 45° | Slight | Free | 0° | Full |
| Seiler et al,[42] 2013 | 4 | NM | Yes | Yes | 0° | NM | 0° | Full |

*Abbreviation:* NM, not mentioned.

fingers are extended. Another example would be that wrist flexion and extension should be performed with the elbow flexed and fingers extended.

### Scar management

Another crucial element of the recovery phase in radial nerve tendon transfers is scar management.[43] Superficial or incisional scars should be managed with scar massage facilitated by lotions and creams that act as lubricants. Other useful adjuncts are silicone gel sheets and pressure stockings to provide compression to the scar. Deep scar management refers to the prevention of tendon adhesions to the surrounding tissue that are detrimental to good tendon gliding and efficient transmission of contractile force.

### Clinical Results and Literature Review

#### Case series and outcomes

The authors present several cases series that have been published over the last 20 years and discuss their outcomes and complications (**Table 6**).[16,24,30,32–34,36,37,44–46] Outcome measures used are fairly heterogeneous, making comparisons between the case series challenging. These physician-rated measures range from strength measurements (grip and pinch) and active range of motion (wrist extension, wrist flexion, finger MCPJ extension, and thumb abduction) to scores dedicated to radial nerve tendon transfers based largely on final range of motion of the wrist and fingers such as those described by Zachary,[28] Chuinard and colleagues,[29] and Bincaz and colleagues.[47] Kapandji's thumb opposition score[48] has also been used in determining functional recovery following these transfers.

#### Complications

Complications for radial nerve tendon transfers in the last 20 years may be summarized as the following (**Table 7**):

1. Limited wrist flexion[30,32,33,44–46]

2. Bowstringing of the PL to EPL transfer[32]
3. Proximal interphalangeal joint flexion contracture when the FDS-type transfer is used[30]
4. Radial deviation when the FCU type is used,[45,46] although some investigators did not encounter this[16,33]
5. Secondary surgery in the form of tenolysis (FCR-type transfer through the interosseous membrane) or cubital tunnel release (FCU-type transfer)[24,32]
6. Wound problems especially when a single incision is used for all transfers[37]
7. Premature fatigue of the hand when either the FCR- or the FCU-type transfer is used[16]

**Donor deficit** One of the principles of tendon transfer is to ensure that the donor muscle is expendable. Particular concern for wrist function has been raised when the FCU is used as a donor tendon because it also participates in DTM.[14] Although investigators have shown that wrist function is retained after FCU transfer[17] and the absence of a PL does not compromise grip and pinch strength,[49] it has been proposed that a functional deficit in forearm pronation occurs after transfer of the PT.[50] As such, due consideration must be given to the latter issue especially in patients whose occupations require strong pronation (eg, for manual laborers consider tendon transfer combinations that do not require the use of the PT with the caveat that these transfers typically use the FCU as a donor; see **Table 3**).[24,36]

### SUMMARY

In this article, the authors have given a broad summary of the available types of radial nerve tendon transfers, a suggested algorithm to help choose the appropriate transfer for an individual patient, the technical tips for a successful procedure, rehabilitation guidelines, and the published outcomes and complications of these transfers. They

---

**Table 5**
**Example of the after-radial nerve tendon transfer rehabilitation program**

| Postoperative Week | Rehabilitation Program |
| --- | --- |
| 0–4 | Immobilization of transfers with mobilization of unaffected joints |
| 4–6 | Protected AROM to gentle PROM and resting splint |
| 6–8 | Muscle retraining and resting splint |
| 8–12 | Muscle strengthening and splint wearing |
| 12 onwards | Full activity |

*Abbreviations:* AROM, active range of motion; PROM, passive range of motion.

**Table 6**
The outcomes reported in recent case series in the past 20 years

| Author, y | Transfer Type | Patient Number | Follow-Up (mo) | Immobilization (wk) | Employment | Patient-Rated Outcome | Physician Rated Outcome | | | | | |
|---|---|---|---|---|---|---|---|---|---|---|---|---|
| | | | | | | | Grip | Pinch | Wrist Extension | Wrist Flexion | Finger MCPJ Extension | Thumb Abduction |
| Dunnet et al,[16] 1995 | FCU/R WAR | 49 | 67 | 3 | NR | NR | 40% | 53% | 22% | NR | 31% (wrist neutral) | NR |
| Kruft et al,[33] 1997 | FCU WAR | 43 | 77 | 3 | 88% | NR | 31 of 29 had a good to very good Zachary score | — | — | — | — | — |
| Skoll et al,[46] 2000 | FCU/R | 22 | 76 | 4 | 76% | NR | 52% | NR | 36% | 34% | 7/22 (wrist extended) | NR |
| Ishida & Ikuta,[32] 2003 | FCR WAR | 21 | 136 | NR | NR | NR | NR | NR | 54° | 42° | 5° (wrist extended) | 36° |
| Ropars et al,[45] 2006 | FCR/FCU | 15 | 114 | 4 | 93% | 13/15 good to excellent (Bincaz) | NR | NR | 38° | 28° | 12/15 (wrist extended) | 54°/8.7 (Kapandji) |
| Gousheh & Arasteh,[24] 2006 | FCU WWR | 108 | 48 | 4 | 92% | NR | 11 kgf | NR | 33° | 52° | 8° (wrist extended) | 38° |
| Krishnan & Schackert,[30] 2008 | FDS | 29 | 33 | 4 | 97% | 4/5 mean patient satisfaction | NR | NR | 46° | NR | 12/29 (wrist extended) | NR |
| Altintas et al,[44] 2009 | FCU/R WAR | 77 | 60 | 3 | 89% | 16 mean DASH | 51% | 70% | 73% | 75% | NR | 80% |
| Chandraprakasam et al,[37] 2009 | FCR | 16 | NR | 4 | NR | NR | NR | NR | NR | NR | NR | NR |
| Monacelli et al,[36] 2011 | FCU WWR | 10 | 12 | 4 | 90% | NR | 11 kgf | NR | 30° | 45° | 8° (wrist extended) | 38° |
| Al-Qattan,[34] 2012 | FCR | 15 | 30 | 5 | 100% | 15/15 good to excellent (Bincaz) | 46% | NR | 45° | 3° | 4° (wrist neutral) | 55°/8.3 (Kapandji) |

Note that results reported as a percentage are compared to the normal side and those reported as degrees is the mean for the sample population.
*Abbreviations:* kgf, kilograms of force; NR, not reported; WAR, with thumb abduction reconstruction; WWR, without dedicated wrist extension reconstruction.

**Table 7**
The complications reported in recent case series in the past 20 years

| Author, y | Transfer Type | Complications | | | | | | |
|---|---|---|---|---|---|---|---|---|
| | | Limited Wrist Flexion | Bowstringing | PIPJ Flexion Contracture | Radial Deviation | Secondary Surgery | Wound Problems | Premature Fatigue |
| Dunnet et al,[16] 1995 | FCU/R WAR | NR | NR | NR | — | NR | NR | ✓ |
| Kruft et al,[33] 1997 | FCU WAR | ✓ | NR | NR | — | NR | NR | NR |
| Skoll et al,[46] 2000 | FCU/R | ✓ | NR | NR | ✓ (FCU used) | NR | NR | NR |
| Ishida & Ikuta,[32] 2003 | FCR WAR | ✓ | ✓ | NR | NR | ✓ | NR | NR |
| Ropars et al,[45] 2006 | FCR/FCU | ✓ | NR | NR | ✓ (FCU used) | NR | NR | NR |
| Gousheh & Arasteh,[24] 2006 | FCU WWR | NR | NR | NR | NR | ✓ | NR | NR |
| Krishnan & Schackert,[30] 2008 | FDS | ✓ | NR | ✓ | NR | NR | ✓ | NR |
| Altintas et al,[44] 2009 | FCU/R WAR | ✓ | NR | NR | NR | NR | NR | NR |
| Chandraprakasam et al,[37] 2009 | FCR | NR | NR | NR | NR | NR | ✓ | NR |
| Monacelli et al,[36] 2011 | FCU WWR | NR | NR | NR | NR | NR | NR | NR |
| Al-Qattan,[34] 2012 | FCR | NR | NR | NR | NR | NR | NR | NR |

*Abbreviations:* NR, not reported; PIPJ, proximal interphalangeal joint; WAR, with thumb abduction reconstruction; WWR, without dedicated wrist extension reconstruction.

reiterate that these transfers must be tailored to each patient and maintain that successful treatment requires first-rate execution of a well-chosen transfer.

## ACKNOWLEDGMENTS

The authors thank Anthony Foo, MD for help in the design of **Fig. 1**.

## REFERENCES

1. Jones NF, Machado GR. Tendon transfers for radial, median, and ulnar nerve injuries: current surgical techniques. Clin Plast Surg 2011;38(4):621–42.
2. Tubiana R, Thomine J, Mackin E. Movements of the hand and wrist. Examination of the hand and wrist. 2nd edition. London: Martin Dunitz; 1996. p. 40–127.
3. Rabischong P. Basic problems in the restoration of prehension. Ann Chir 1971;25(19):927–33 [in French].
4. Burkhalter WE. Early tendon transfer in upper extremity peripheral nerve injury. Clin Orthop Relat Res 1974;(104):68–79.
5. Lowe JB 3rd, Sen SK, Mackinnon SE. Current approach to radial nerve paralysis. Plast Reconstr Surg 2002;110(4):1099–113.
6. Ratner JA, Peljovich A, Kozin SH. Update on tendon transfers for peripheral nerve injuries. J Hand Surg Am 2010;35(8):1371–81.
7. Tsuge K. Tendon transfers for radial nerve palsy. Aust N Z J Surg 1980;50(3):267–72.
8. Sammer DM, Chung KC. Tendon transfers: part I. Principles of transfer and transfers for radial nerve palsy. Plast Reconstr Surg 2009;123(5):169e–77e.
9. Lieber RL, Jacobson MD, Fazeli BM, et al. Architecture of selected muscles of the arm and forearm: anatomy and implications for tendon transfer. J Hand Surg Am 1992;17(5):787–98.
10. Boyes JH. Selection of a donor muscle for tendon transfer. Bull Hosp Joint Dis 1962;23:1–4.
11. Brand PW, Beach RB, Thompson DE. Relative tension and potential excursion of muscles in the forearm and hand. J Hand Surg Am 1981;6(3):209–19.
12. Smith RJ. Tendon transfers of the hand and forearm. Boston: Little Brown; 1987.
13. Moritomo H, Apergis EP, Garcia-Elias M, et al. International Federation of Societies for Surgery of the Hand 2013 Committee's report on wrist dart-throwing motion. J Hand Surg Am 2014;39(7):1433–9.
14. Werner FW, Short WH, Palmer AK, et al. Wrist tendon forces during various dynamic wrist motions. J Hand Surg Am 2010;35(4):628–32.
15. Green D. Radial nerve palsy. In: Green D, Hotchkiss R, Pederson W, et al, editors. Operative hand surgery, vol. 2, 5th edition. New York: Churchill Livingstone; 2005. p. 1113–31.
16. Dunnet WJ, Housden PL, Birch R. Flexor to extensor tendon transfers in the hand. J Hand Surg Br 1995;20(1):26–8.
17. Raskin KB, Wilgis EF. Flexor carpi ulnaris transfer for radial nerve palsy: functional testing of long-term results. J Hand Surg Am 1995;20(5):737–42.
18. Sebastin SJ, Puhaindran ME, Lim AY, et al. The prevalence of absence of the palmaris longus–a study in a Chinese population and a review of the literature. J Hand Surg Br 2005;30(5):525–7.
19. Brand PW. Tendon transfers in the forearm. In: Flynn JE, editor. Hand surgery. 2nd edition. Baltimore (MA): Williams and Wilkins; 1975. p. 189–200.
20. Merle d'Aubigne R. Treatment of residual paralysis after injuries of the main nerves; superior extremity. Proc R Soc Med 1949;42(10):831–5. illust.
21. Riordan DC. Tendon transfers in hand surgery. J Hand Surg Am 1983;8(5 Pt 2):748–53.
22. Brooks DM. Tendon transfer for paralysis. In: Birch R, Brooks DM, editors. Rob and Smith's operative surgery: the hand. London: Butterworths; 1984. p. 310–4.
23. Lim AY, Lahiri A, Pereira BP, et al. Independent function in a split flexor carpi radialis transfer. J Hand Surg Am 2004;29(1):28–31.
24. Gousheh J, Arasteh E. Transfer of a single flexor carpi ulnaris tendon for treatment of radial nerve palsy. J Hand Surg Br 2006;31(5):542–6.
25. Jones R. II. On suture of nerves, and alternative methods of treatment by transplantation of tendon. Br Med J 1916;1(2889):679–82.
26. Said GZ. A modified tendon transference for radial nerve paralysis. J Bone Joint Surg Br 1974;56(2):320–2.
27. Tubiana R. Problems and solutions in palliative tendon transfer surgery for radial nerve palsy. Tech Hand Up Extrem Surg 2002;6(3):104–13.
28. Zachary RB. Tendon transplantation for radial paralysis. Br J Surg 1946;34:358–64.
29. Chuinard RG, Boyes JH, Stark HH, et al. Tendon transfers for radial nerve palsy: use of superficialis tendons for digital extension. J Hand Surg Am 1978;3(6):560–70.
30. Krishnan KG, Schackert G. An analysis of results after selective tendon transfers through the interosseous membrane to provide selective finger and thumb extension in chronic irreparable radial nerve lesions. J Hand Surg Am 2008;33(2):223–31.
31. Starr CL. Army experiences with tendon transference. J Bone Joint Surg Am 1922;3:3–21.
32. Ishida O, Ikuta Y. Analysis of Tsuge's procedure for the treatment of radial nerve paralysis. Hand Surg 2003;8(1):17–20.
33. Kruft S, von Heimburg D, Reill P. Treatment of irreversible lesion of the radial nerve by tendon transfer: indication and long-term results of the Merle

d'Aubigne procedure. Plast Reconstr Surg 1997; 100(3):610–6 [discussion: 617–8].

34. Al-Qattan MM. Tendon transfer for radial nerve palsy: a single tendon to restore finger extension as well as thumb extension/radial abduction. J Hand Surg Eur Vol 2012;37(9):855–62.

35. Jones R. II. On suture of nerves, and alternative methods of treatment by transplantation of tendon. Br Med J 1916;1(2888):641–3.

36. Monacelli G, Spagnoli AM, Rizzo MI, et al. Treatment of persistent radial nerve palsy through "tendon minimal transfer" technique. G Chir 2011;32(1–2):69–72.

37. Chandraprakasam T, Gavaskar AS, Prabhakaran T. Modified Jones transfer for radial nerve palsy using a single incision: surgical technique. Tech Hand Up Extrem Surg 2009;13(1):16–8.

38. Colantoni Woodside J, Bindra RR. Rerouting extensor pollicis longus tendon transfer. J Hand Surg Am 2015;40(4):822–5.

39. Brooks DM. Tendon transplantation in the forearm and arthrodesis of the wrist. Proc R Soc Med 1949; 42(10):838–43.

40. Peljovich A, Ratner JA, Marino J. Update of the physiology and biomechanics of tendon transfer surgery. J Hand Surg Am 2010;35(8):1365–9 [quiz: 1370].

41. Friden J, Lieber RL. Evidence for muscle attachment at relatively long lengths in tendon transfer surgery. J Hand Surg Am 1998;23(1):105–10.

42. Seiler JG 3rd, Desai MJ, Payne SH. Tendon transfers for radial, median, and ulnar nerve palsy. J Am Acad Orthop Surg 2013;21(11):675–84.

43. Kozin SH. Tendon transfers for radial and median nerve palsies. J Hand Ther 2005;18(2):208–15.

44. Altintas AA, Altintas MA, Gazyakan E, et al. Long-term results and the disabilities of the arm, shoulder, and hand score analysis after modified Brooks and D'Aubigne tendon transfer for radial nerve palsy. J Hand Surg Am 2009;34(3):474–8.

45. Ropars M, Dreano T, Siret P, et al. Long-term results of tendon transfers in radial and posterior interosseous nerve paralysis. J Hand Surg Br 2006;31(5): 502–6.

46. Skoll PJ, Hudson DA, de Jager W, et al. Long-term results of tendon transfers for radial nerve palsy in patients with limited rehabilitation. Ann Plast Surg 2000;45(2):122–6.

47. Bincaz LE, Cherifi H, Alnot JY. Palliative tendon transfer for reanimation of the wrist and finger extension lag. Report of 14 transfers for radial nerve palsies and ten transfers for brachial plexus lesions. Chir Main 2002;21(1):13–22 [in French].

48. Kapandji A. Clinical test of apposition and counter-apposition of the thumb. Ann Chir Main 1986;5(1): 67–73 [in French].

49. Sebastin SJ, Lim AY, Bee WH, et al. Does the absence of the palmaris longus affect grip and pinch strength? J Hand Surg Br 2005;30(4):406–8.

50. Skie MC, Parent TE, Mudge KM, et al. Functional deficit after transfer of the pronator teres for acquired radial nerve palsy. J Hand Surg Am 2007; 32(4):526–30.

# High Median Nerve Injuries

Jonathan Isaacs, MD[a],*, Obinna Ugwu-Oju, MD[b]

## KEYWORDS

- High median nerve palsy • Nerve injuries • Tendon transfers

## KEY POINTS

- High median nerve injuries are defined as lesions proximal to the takeoff of the anterior interosseous nerve.
- Opposition, thumb flexion, flexion of the index and middle fingers, and pronation may suffer variable functional deficits.
- Thumb flexion may be restored using a well-mobilized brachioradialis tendon transfer.
- Index and middle finger flexion are most commonly addressed via a side-to-side tendon transfer with the tendons of the small and ring flexor digitorum profundus.

## INTRODUCTION

The median nerve serves a crucial role in extrinsic and intrinsic motor and sensory function to the radial half of the hand. High median nerve injuries, defined as injuries proximal to the anterior interosseous nerve origin, therefore typically result in significant functional loss prompting aggressive surgical management. Even with appropriate recognition and contemporary nerve reconstruction, however, motor and sensory recovery may be inadequate. With isolated persistent high median nerve palsies, a variety of available tendon transfers can improve key motor functions and salvage acceptable use of the hand.

## NATURE OF THE PROBLEM

The median nerve is vulnerable to direct penetrating trauma owing to gunshot, knife, or broken glass, as common examples, throughout its course. Fractures of the distal humerus can stretch or avulse the nerve in both adults and children,[1,2] and less commonly the nerve may become incarcerated in a reduced fracture or elbow

dislocation.[3] Median nerve entrapment in a distal humerus fracture can be suspected when an ulnar cortical indentation in the distal humeral metaphysis is noted on the anteroposterior radiograph, also known as a "Matev sign."[4] Acute compressive damage associated with unrecognized or undertreated hematoma formation has been noted after brachial artery catheterization,[5] and median nerve injury has been reported rarely as an elbow arthroscopy complication.[6,7] Perhaps one of the most frustrating iatrogenic causes of high median nerve damage that we have seen is from overzealous traction or careless positioning of self-retaining retractors during a variety of surgical procedures.[8]

## ANATOMY

The median nerve receives contributions from all 5 roots of the brachial plexus via the lateral and medial cords and passes down the medial arm between the biceps brachii and brachialis muscles, intimately parallel with the brachial artery. As the nerve descends, it moves from a lateral to a more anterior relationship to traverse

[a] Division of Hand Surgery, Department of Orthopaedic Surgery, Virginia Commonwealth University Health System, 1200 E Broad Street, Richmond, VA 23298, USA; [b] Department of Orthopaedic Surgery, Virginia Commonwealth University Health System, 1200 E Broad Street, Richmond, VA 23298, USA
* Corresponding author.
E-mail address: jonathan.isaacs@vcuhealth.org

Hand Clin 32 (2016) 339–348
http://dx.doi.org/10.1016/j.hcl.2016.03.004
0749-0712/16/$ – see front matter © 2016 Elsevier Inc. All rights reserved.

the antecubital fossa, pass between the 2 heads of the pronator teres, and continue to the hand between the flexor digitorum superficialis and profundus muscle bellies. The anterior interosseous nerve, the largest and only branch to take off the radial side of the median nerve, originates on average 5.4 cm distal to the medial epicondyle to innervate the flexor digitorum profundus (FDP) to the index and middle fingers, the flexor pollicus longus (FPL), and the pronator quadratus.[9] Separate branches of the median nerve in the proximal forearm innervate the pronator teres, the flexor digitorum superficialis, the flexor carpi radialis, and the palmaris longus (if present). An anatomic study by Bhadra and colleagues[10] showed dual innervation of the long finger FDP by the anterior interosseous nerve and ulnar nerves in 75% of specimens, and 5% of specimens solely had ulnar innervation. Proximal to the wrist, the palmar cutaneous branch arborizes before the median nerve continues through the carpal tunnel to provide terminal innervation to the index and middle lumbricals, and the thenar muscles, as well as supplying sensation to the radial 3.5 digits.

Untreated or persistent high median nerve palsies, therefore, affect forearm pronation, finger flexion, thumb flexion, wrist flexion, and thumb opposition. When the injury is confined to the median nerve, redundant motor function from ulnar-innervated muscles maintain adequate wrist flexion (through the flexor carpi ulnaris), and ring and little finger flexion (through the ulnar side of the FDP) so that the residual extrinsic functional losses include lack of forearm pronation, and index finger, middle finger, and thumb flexion. Although the flexor carpi radialis, palmaris longus, and flexor digitorum superficialis (specifically to the ring finger) are functionally not "missed," they are no longer available as potential opponensplasty donor tendons (see Gaston RG, Chadderdon RC: Low Median Nerve Transfers (Opponensplasty), in this issue). The loss of sensation, especially along the opposing surfaces of the thumb and index finger, can be particularly disruptive and should be addressed regardless of motor reconstruction strategy.

High median nerve palsy discrepancies have been reported and can most easily be explained by abnormal anatomic connections between the ulnar and median nerve distal to the elbow. Patients with Martin–Gruber anastomoses lose traditionally ulnar-innervated intrinsic function with high median injury. In rare reports of Riche–Cannieu or ulnar-to-median innervation, thenar musculature may retain function in the setting of proximal median nerve insult. Pure sensory anastomoses, including Marinacci and Berretini anastomoses, also need to be considered with seemingly "nonanatomic" loss of sensation after injury.[11]

The functional significance of forearm pronation loss has been debated in the literature. Bertelli and colleagues[12] argues that this function is typically not completely lost and is of low priority. In his series of 11 high median nerve injuries, however, strong pronation was preserved through a more limited arc in almost all patients (the 1 patient without pronation had a concomitant elbow fracture). A variety of muscles, including the brachialis, the FDP, and the extensor carpi ulnaris, perhaps working in concert, seem to be capable of compensating for the denervated pronators. Gravity, combined with shoulder abduction and internal rotation, can affectively position the forearm in pronation as well. MacKinnon and colleagues,[13] conversely, emphasize the importance of this function and encourage aggressive efforts at restoring active pronation. Our experience suggests that some patients are able to compensate and others are not. However, the importance of being able to place the forearm in a pronated position (either using the shoulder or active forearm pronation) is obvious. Writing, typing, and eating all require hand pronation.[14,15] The need to surgically reestablish active pronation must be, therefore, individualized for each patient.

Middle finger flexion is not always affected, either owing to either crossover innervation from the ulnar nerve (to the FDP to the middle finger) or from more tenacious soft tissue connections between the middle and ring FDP muscles. No patient in Bertelli's series lacked middle finger FDP flexion strength.[12] Loss of isolated FPL function can be treated adequately with interphalangeal joint arthrodesis, but is a more significant problem when combined with loss of thenar muscle function.[16] The combined loss of thumb, index, and middle finger flexion negatively impacts gross pinch and grip as well as finer dexterity maneuvers, including typing and manipulating smaller objects.

## SURGICAL TECHNIQUE
### Preoperative Planning

Although most surgeons would recommend exploration and primary repair or reconstruction as part of the initial management for most obvious median nerve injuries, poor clinical predictability in many situations may hamper this enthusiasm. Muscle reinnervation must occur within a limited window of opportunity (of around 18 months after injury). Even with spontaneous axonal regeneration (after axonotometic injury) or acute repair, prolonged denervation is inevitable owing to protracted regeneration times associated with very proximal injuries.[17] This already tenuous situation is exacerbated with delayed presentation or prolonged "observation" periods. Large zones of injury, unfavorable tissue beds at the proposed nerve repair site, and advanced patient age are other negative prognostic factors that must be considered. Only 10% of proximal median nerve repairs achieved successful recovery in 1 study, and a metaanalysis of major peripheral nerve repairs in the upper extremity reported desirable outcomes only around 50% of the time.[18,19] Sensory recovery is less time sensitive than motor recovery, and proximal repair may still be performed with this more limited goal combined with planned tendon transfers.

The timing for tendon transfer, therefore, must be individualized and based on expected recovery. With a low chance of motor recovery (related to prolonged period of denervation, devastating injury, or patient characteristics), early tendon transfer would be indicated. A patient of ours suffered an incomplete above elbow arm amputation with a relatively isolated median nerve injury. Although he was young and otherwise a good candidate for nerve repair, the zone of injury included an arterial reconstruction and had been skin grafted, and the initial median nerve loss was estimated at 15 to 20 cm (**Fig. 1**). The decision was made to turn directly to tendon transfers without attempting the potentially morbid and unpredictable nerve reconstruction.

For patients in whom potential spontaneous axonal regeneration may still occur or median nerve repair has been performed with the intent of reinnervation, adequate time for recovery based on at least a 1-inch per month nerve regeneration rate (plus a 3-month buffer) is typically respected

before secondary reconstructive options are considered. Unlike some other nerve palsies, however, the donor and recipient tendons are closely approximated so that proximal release of the recipient tendons is not always necessary. This means that early transfer (using donor to "side" of intact recipient tendon) allows maintenance of the recipient motor/tendon unit and does not necessarily "burn bridges" if eventual reinnervation were to occur. For example, the brachioradialis can be transferred to the side of the intact FPL without releasing the FPL proximally to achieve functional thumb flexion. If eventually the FPL is reanimated, this added muscle power will only augment thumb pinch strength. In either case, as with all tendon transfers, the soft tissue envelope must be stable, proposed donor tendons must be functional, and the paralyzed components of the upper extremity must be supple before proceeding. Regaining some level of sensory function will clearly maximize the functional usefulness of any tendon transfers and, in cases of persistent anesthesia, nerve transfers should be considered in conjunction with the tendon reconstruction (**Fig. 2**).

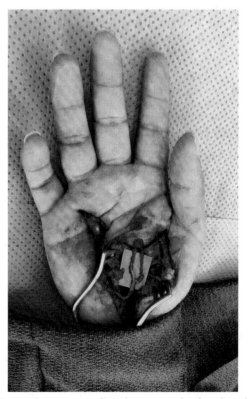

Fig. 2. The common digital nerve to the fourth web space being transferred to the radial digital nerve of the index and the ulnar digital nerve of the thumb to restore critical sensation to the border digits of the first web space.

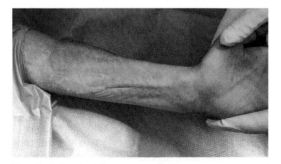

Fig. 1. Patient status post soft tissue coverage and bony repair of partial arm amputation. Owing to an unfavorable tissue bed and large median nerve defect, his functional deficits were addressed using a sensory nerve transfer and brachioradialis to flexor pollicus longus and flexor digitorum profundus side-to-side tendon transfers.

Staging and the order of procedures are somewhat controversial. In general, if pronation is restored first, then rehabilitating the fingers/thumb will be easier because the patient will more easily incorporate their usage into daily activities. However, the forearm must be at least passively supinated to gain access to the FPL and FDP tendons (if this is performed as a secondary surgery). Conversely, if finger/thumb flexion (and thumb opposition) is addressed initially, the patient may still struggle placing the hand into a position where these transfers can be best appreciated. Doing both procedures simultaneously may result in excessive hand swelling and mobilizing transferred tendons for the digits conflicts with the protective immobilization after pronation transfers.

Common transfers are straightforward and typically available for most high median nerve injuries and include:

- Brachioradialis to FPL;
- Ring and little FDP side-to-side transfer to index and/or middle FDP; and
- Biceps rerouting around proximal radius to convert direction of biceps tendon pull to a pronating force.

In rare circumstances alternative transfers that may be useful:

- Extensor carpi radialis brevis (ECRB) to FPL; and
- Extensor carpi radialis longus (ECRL) to FDP (index and middle).

### Preparation and Patient Positioning

- Patient should be placed supine on the operating table with the arm abducted 90° onto a hand board. If a biceps tendon transfer is planned, then the brachium should be prepped in and a sterile tourniquet used. Otherwise, a proximal nonsterile tourniquet is appropriate.
- Either regional or general anesthesia can be established.
- Prepping and draping should leave the elbow free and include the brachium (for pronation transfers).

## SURGICAL APPROACH

Thumb interphalangeal flexion and index and middle FDP reanimation can be achieved through the same incision.

- The incision starts at the wrist flexion crease and is carried proximally over the flexor carpi radialis tendon about two-thirds the length of the forearm (**Fig. 3**).

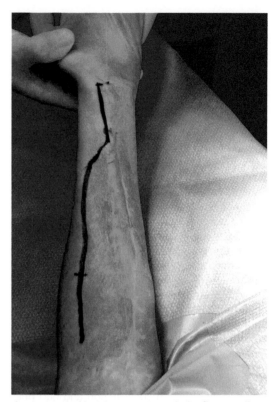

**Fig. 3.** Surgical incision to approach the flexor pollicus longus, brachioradialis, and flexor digitorum profundus tendons. The incision in this patient was brought a little more radial than normal to accommodate the skin grafted area in his forearm but is carried quite proximal to allow adequate mobilization of the brachioradialis.

- The superficial fascia is incised in line with the flexor carpi radialis tendon, which is than mobilized and retracted.
- The floor of the flexor carpi radialis tendon is incised the length of the incision (and released several centimeters proximal to the skin incision) and blunt dissection used to expose the deep tissues (the pronator quadratus) in the distal forearm.
- The FPL is identified deep to the flexor carpi radialis and superficial to the pronator quadratus (**Fig. 4**). The 4 tendons of the FDP are located just superficial to the pronator quadratus and ulnar to the FPL (**Fig. 5**).
- The brachioradialis can be identified inserting into the radial styloid and is approached deep to the radial artery, which is retracted radially.

Alternative approach when using ECRL or ECRB

- The volar incision can be shifted more radially b it is extended proximally if the brachioradialis still needs to be dissected free, but the

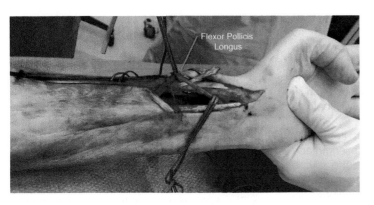

**Fig. 4.** The flexor pollicus longus has been isolated deep to the flexor carpi radialis tendon.

ECRL can still be reached in the mid forearm by dissecting in a subcutaneous plane around the radial border.

- If the brachioradialis is not to be used at all, the donor ECRL and ECRB tendons and the FPL and FDP (index and/or middle) recipient tendons can be exposed via a second mid radial incision.
- A small additional transverse incision may be necessary at the ECRL (and/or ECRB) insertion sites at the radial base of the index (and/or middle) metacarpal(s) (although this area may be exposed by dissecting around the radial border of the wrist).

The biceps tendon is exposed at the antecubital fossa and the proximal forearm.

- An approximately 15-cm serpentine incision is made starting medially and extending distally and obliquely across the antecubital fossa before continuing distally lateral to the biceps tendon.
- After cutting through skin, the cephalic vein and venous system needs to be dissected free and mobilized. Although some branches can be tied off, the larger veins should be preserved. The lateral antebrachial cutaneous

nerve should be identified in the lateral aspect of the surgical exposure and preserved.
- Beware of the brachial artery and median nerve just medial to the biceps tendon and the radial nerve crossing the elbow between the proximal brachioradialis muscle and the distal brachialis muscles.
- The intervals between the brachioradialis and the brachialis (proximal) and between the brachioradialis and the pronator teres (distal) should be developed.
- The thick fascia known as the lacertus fibrosis overlying the biceps tendon is incised and the tendon exposed.

## SURGICAL PROCEDURE

Thumb interphalangeal flexion
- The BR is sharply lifted away from its insertion on the radial styloid and is dissected proximally at least three-fourth of the way up the forearm to adequately mobilize it. There is a mismatch between the excursion of the FPL and the brachioradialis, and this can be partially compensated by extensive brachioradialis tendon/muscle mobilization and release from surrounding tissues. Once adequately

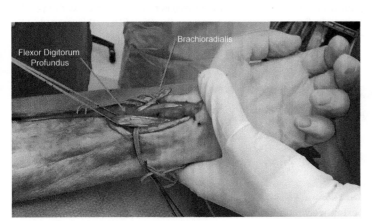

**Fig. 5.** The flexor digitorum profundus has been isolated between the pronator quadratus and the flexor digitorum superficialis tendons. The brachioradialis tendon has been sharply released from its insertion into the radial styloid.

mobilized, the brachioradialis should have at least 3 cm of excursion[20](**Fig. 6**).

- The FPL is released at the muscle tendon junction, which typically gives abundant tendon for transfer. Alternatively, if there is the potential still for delayed reinnervation of the FPL muscle, the brachioradialis can be transferred to the side of the FPL without proximal release. With the wrist in neutral, the brachioradialis is pulled out to length and the FPL pulled proximally (with the thumb flexed). The elbow should be at approximately 45° of flexion because the brachioradialis originates above the elbow.
- The brachioradialis tendon is broad and flat and can be laid alongside or wrapped around the FPL tendon. Two to 3 horizontal mattress "stay sutures" (using 3-0 braided suture material) should be placed across the overlapping tendons before checking the tension with a tenodesis test.
- The tension is judged based on wrist position. The thumb should be fully extendable with the wrist flexed (**Fig. 7**A) and should flex fully with the wrist extended (**Fig. 7**B). If the tension is not appropriate, the "stay sutures" should be carefully removed (a #15 blade to cut out the knot works well), and revised until the tension is correct.
- Once the tension is correctly dialed in, the tendon transfer is completed by running a 4-0 braided suture up and down 1 edge of the overlapping tendons (should be ≥3 cm). The goal is to take several small tissue bites and to smooth the interface between the 2 tendons. The suture can be tied back to its starting point and, when complete, should look like a running "baseball" stitch. This is repeated on the opposite overlapping edges so that the final repair consists of 2 to 3 "stay sutures" and 2 rows of running "crisscross" stitches the length of the overlapping tendons (**Fig. 8**).
- Alternatively, the brachioradialis tendon can be weaved through 2 "stab" incisions in line with but on perpendicular surfaces of the FPL tendon (as described by Pulvertaft[21]).

Tension is set the same as described, and the woven tendons secured with several small sutures.

- The side-to-side technique is stronger and stiffer than the Pulvertaft tendon weave[19,22] and is our preferred technique. In our experience, the Pulvertaft-type weaves tend to be more bulky and if "readjustments" of the tension are necessary, the tendons tend to become frayed and untidy.

Index and middle flexion
- The FDP tendons of the index and middle fingers are pulled proximally so that these 2 fingers cascade into a slightly greater flexion than the ring and little digits.
- While maintaining this alignment, 3 or 4 horizontal mattress sutures are placed across all 4 FDP tendons (using 2-0 braided suture material; **Fig. 9**). The goal is to have all 4 fingers flex together.

Alternative transfers
- After releasing the ECRL (and/or ECRB) at their insertion sites, the tendons are withdrawn proximally until they can be transferred in a straight line to the FPL and FDP tendons.
- If both the index and middle FDP tendons are transferred together (the middle may not require transfer), they can be sutured side-to-side to be transferred as a "single unit."
- The FPL and FDP tendon(s) are cut proximally at the muscle tendon junction and swung toward the ECRL (and/or ECRB) tendons, which are passed in a subcutaneous plane around the radial border of the forearm.
- The overlapping tendons are sutured together (typically ECRL to FDP and/or ECRB to FPL). Tension should be set such that the fingers/thumb flex with the wrist extended and can be extended passively with the wrist flexed. Because there is more excursion with the FDP compared with the FPL, this should be tensioned first and the index (and/or middle) digits should cascade into a slightly tighter fist

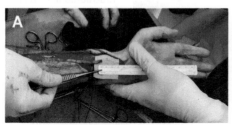
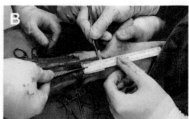

**Fig. 6.** (A) The brachioradialis has been extensively mobilized. (B) Demonstrating 3 cm of excurcison.

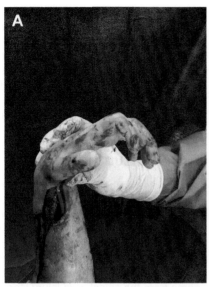
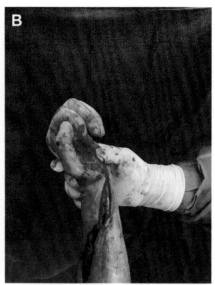

**Fig. 7.** After proper tension of the tendon transfers, (*A*) the fingers and thumb extend with passive wrist flexion and (*B*) flexion of the digits with passive wrist extension.

than the other digits. The FPL transfer should err on being a little looser than the FDP transfer, but care must be taken with both so as to not create an iatrogenic flexion contracture.
- Typically, if one of the wrist extensors is to be used, the ECRL is transferred to increase index/middle flexion strength and the brachioradialis is still transferred to the FPL.

Biceps rerouting for pronation
- The biceps tendon is followed down to its insertion of the radius and isolated. The tendon and muscle can be mobilized proximally. Using the entire length of the biceps tendon, it is cut in a z-plasty pattern.

- A plane is made around the lateral aspect of the radial neck (take care to not damage the radial nerve running approximately 8 mm from the radiocapitellar joint.[23] A plane is made around the medial aspect and a right angle hemostat used to create a path completely around the radial neck. Alternatively supinating and pronating the forearm will help with access and visualization.
- Once the plane is established, the distal tendon stump is passed medially and posteriorly around the radial neck and brought back into the operative field around the lateral aspect of the radial neck. Sutures can be placed into the stump to assist in this rerouting and their passage can be facilitated using a right angle hemostat or by contouring a suture passer.

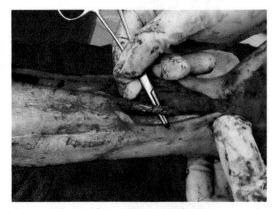

**Fig. 8.** Side-to-side tendon transfer between the brachioradialis and the flexor pollicus longus. Note the running "crisscross" stitches up both edges of the overlapping tendons.

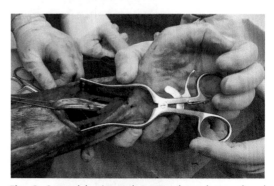

**Fig. 9.** Several horizontal sutures have been placed across the flexor digitorum profundus tendons to create a side-to-side transfer.

- With the forearm pronated fully, the overlapping biceps tendon stumps can be sutured side-to-side over as much distance as possible. Based on the average circumference of the radial neck, 1.5 cm of tendon length is typically lost.[24]

## IMMEDIATE POSTOPERATIVE CARE

Biceps rerouting
- The elbow is immobilized for 4 weeks at 90° of flexion and maximum pronation.
- At 4 weeks, the forearm is allowed to supinate to neutral and gentle passive range of motion of the elbow and forearm is initiated. A sugar tong splint is used when not performing rehabilitative exercises.
- At 6 weeks, full range of motion is allowed and gentle strengthening initiated.
- At 3 months, unrestricted activity is allowed.

Brachioradialis to FPL and side-to-side FDP transfers (and ECRL/ECRB transfers)
- Postoperatively, the hand is placed in a safe position with the MCP joints flexed and the interphalangeal joints in neutral. The thumb is held with a thumb spica extension to the splint. The wrist is flexed approximately 30° to take tension off of the repairs (or in neutral if ECRL/ECRB are used).
- At 2 weeks, the hand/wrist are placed in a removable safe position dorsal hand splint (with thumb spica extension). The splint is

removed for gentle active/passive assist range of motion using wrist tenodesis effect.
- The splint is worn when not doing rehabilitative exercises until 6 weeks postoperatively. At that time, strengthening exercises are initiated and a gradual return to normal activities allowed.
- Unrestricted activity is allowed at 3 months postoperatively (**Fig. 10**).

## CLINICAL RESULTS

Few studies describe long-term results for tendon transfers for high median nerve injuries and it is difficult to separate out functional improvement specifically from motor reanimation versus sensory restoration. Indeed, most clinical outcomes studies focus on the sensory aspect,[25] so that some of our data on these transfers must come from the spinal cord injury literature.

Considered reliable and straightforward for high median nerve injuries, side-to-side FDP transfers have been shown to restore synchronization and force distribution between fingers in tetraplegics.[26,27] Likewise, 15 of 17 partially paralyzed hands had improvement with restoration of pinch with the brachioradialis to FPL transfer.[28] In a smaller series, 4 of 5 patients made gains with the brachioradialis to FPL transfer.[29]

Even less commonly reported is the use of tendon transfers for the restoration of pronation in the adult population. This may be related to Bertelli and colleague's[12] observation that

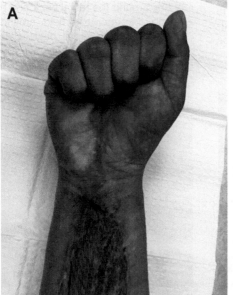
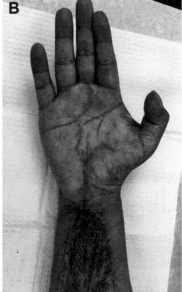

**Fig. 10.** Healed tendon transfers for high median nerve injury demonstrating (*A*) excellent index and middle digit flexion and (*B*) excellent thumb interphalangeal flexion.

pronation is more of a theoretic loss than an actual clinical problem after high median nerve injuries. Zancolli[30] initially described the biceps rerouting procedure for birth palsy, traumatic quadriplegia, and poliomyelitis. After this, a larger study by Owings and colleagues[31] reported largely good and satisfactory results in patients, with some loss of supination as the only common negative finding. Results in adult patients in the setting of tetraplegia have also shown improvement in the amount of pronation, specifically in Gellman's cohort of 8 limbs in 6 tetraplegic patients, increasing pronation by 75° with biceps rerouting.[32]

## SUMMARY

Median nerve reconstruction or sensory nerve transfer combined with (most commonly) brachioradialis to FPL and side-to-side FDP tendon transfers can provide consistent and substantial functional improvement in patients suffering high median nerve injury.

## REFERENCES

1. Rohilla R, Singla R, Magu N-K, et al. Combined radial and median nerve injury in diaphyseal fracture of humerus: a case report. Chin J Traumatol 2013; 16(6):365–7.

2. Dormans JP, Squillante R, Sharf H. Acute neurovascular complications with supracondylar humerus fractures in children. J Hand Surg 1995;20(1):1–4.

3. Simon D, Masquijo JJ, Duncan MJ, et al. Intra-articular median nerve incarceration after spontaneous reduction of a pediatric elbow dislocation: case report and review of the literature. J Pediatr Orthop 2010;30(2):125–9.

4. Matev I. A radiological sign of entrapment of the median nerve in the elbow joint after posterior dislocation. A report of two cases. J Bone Joint Surg Br 1976;58(3):353–5.

5. Kennedy AM, Grocott M, Schwartz MS, et al. Median nerve injury: an underrecognised complication of brachial artery cardiac catheterisation? J Neurol Neurosurg Psychiatry 1997;63(4):542–6.

6. Haapaniemi T, Berggren M, Adolfsson L. Complete transection of the median and radial nerves during arthroscopic release of post-traumatic elbow contracture. Arthroscopy 1999;15(7):784–7.

7. Adams JE, Steinmann SP. Nerve injuries about the elbow. J Hand Surg 2006;31(2):303–13.

8. Winfree CJ, Kline DG. Intraoperative positioning nerve injuries. Surg Neurol 2005;63(1):5–18 [discussion: 18].

9. Tubbs RS, Custis JW, Salter EG, et al. Quantitation of and superficial surgical landmarks for the anterior interosseous nerve. J Neurosurg 2006; 104(5):787–91.

10. Bhadra N, Keith MW, Peckham PH. Variations in innervation of the flexor digitorum profundus muscle. J Hand Surg 1999;24(4):700–3.

11. Dogan NU, Uysal II, Seker M. The communications between the ulnar and median nerves in upper limb. Neuroanatomy 2009;8:20–5.

12. Bertelli JA, Soldado F, Lehn VLM, et al. Reappraisal of Clinical deficits following high median nerve injuries. J Hand Surg 2016;41(1):13–9.

13. Hsiao EC, Fox IK, Tung TH, et al. Motor nerve transfers to restore extrinsic median nerve function: case report. Hand 2009;4(1):92–7.

14. Morrey BF, Askew LJ, Chao EY. A biomechanical study of normal functional elbow motion. J Bone Joint Surg Am 1981;63(6):872–7.

15. Sardelli M, Tashjian RZ, MacWilliams BA. Functional elbow range of motion for contemporary tasks. J Bone Joint Surg Am 2011;93(5):471–7.

16. Colyer RA, Kappelman B. Flexor pollicis longus tenodesis in tetraplegia at the sixth cervical level. A prospective evaluation of functional gain. J Bone Joint Surg Am 1981;63(3):376–9.

17. Isaacs J. Major peripheral nerve injuries. Hand Clin 2013;29(3):371–82.

18. Roganovic Z. Missile-caused median nerve injuries: results of 81 repairs. Surg Neurol 2005;63(5):410–8 [discussion: 418–9].

19. Ruijs ACJ, Jaquet J-B, Kalmijn S, et al. Median and ulnar nerve injuries: a meta-analysis of predictors of motor and sensory recovery after modern microsurgical nerve repair. Plast Reconstr Surg 2005;116(2): 484–94 [discussion: 495–6].

20. Fridén J, Albrecht D, Lieber RL. Biomechanical analysis of the brachioradialis as a donor in tendon transfer. Clin Orthop Relat Res 2001;(383):152–61.

21. Pulvertaft RG. Tendon grafts for flexor tendon injuries in the fingers and thumb; a study of technique and results. J Bone Joint Surg Br 1956; 38-B(1):175–94.

22. Brown SHM, Hentzen ER, Kwan A, et al. Mechanical strength of the side-to-side versus Pulvertaft weave tendon repair. J Hand Surg 2010;35(4):540–5.

23. Hackl M, Lappen S, Burkhart KJ, et al. The course of the median and radial nerve across the elbow: an anatomic study. Arch Orthop Trauma Surg 2015; 135(7):979–83.

24. Manske PR, McCarroll HR, Hale R. Biceps tendon rerouting and percutaneous osteoclasis in the treatment of supination deformity in obstetrical palsy. J Hand Surg 1980;5(2):153–9.

25. Burkhalter WE. Early tendon transfer in upper extremity peripheral nerve injury. Clin Orthop Relat Res 1974;(104):68–79.

26. Keith MW, Kilgore KL, Peckham PH, et al. Tendon transfers and functional electrical stimulation for

restoration of hand function in spinal cord injury. J Hand Surg 1996;21(1):89–99.

27. Keith MW, Peckham PH, Thrope GB, et al. Functional neuromuscular stimulation neuroprostheses for the tetraplegic hand. Clin Orthop Relat Res 1988;(233):25–33.

28. Waters R, Moore KR, Graboff SR, et al. Brachioradialis to flexor pollicis longus tendon transfer for active lateral pinch in the tetraplegic. J Hand Surg 1985; 10(3):385–91.

29. Failla JM, Peimer CA, Sherwin FS. Brachioradialis transfer for digital palsy. J Hand Surg Br 1990; 15(3):312–6.

30. Zancolli EA. Paralytic supination contracture of the forearm. J Bone Joint Surg Am 1967;49(7): 1275–84.

31. Owings R, Wickstrom J, Perry J, et al. Biceps brachii rerouting in treatment of paralytic supination contracture of the forearm. J Bone Joint Surg Am 1971;53(1):137–42.

32. Gellman H, Kan D, Waters RL, et al. Rerouting of the biceps brachii for paralytic supination contracture of the forearm in tetraplegia due to trauma. J Bone Joint Surg Am 1994;76(3):398–402.

# Low Median Nerve Transfers (Opponensplasty)

Robert Christopher Chadderdon, MD,
R. Glenn Gaston, MD*

## KEYWORDS

- Opponensplasty • Opposition • Tendon transfer • Camitz • Huber • Pinch

## KEY POINTS

- Thumb opposition is a combination of flexion, palmar abduction, and pronation.
- The abductor pollicis brevis (APB) is the most important muscle in thumb opposition, and reanimating its function and line of pull should be the goal of tendon transfers for restoration of opposition.
- The palmaris longus is frequently chosen as a donor to restore palmar abduction of the thumb when chronic median nerve compression is the cause and carpal tunnel release is being performed.
- The flexor digitorum superficialis tendon can be used effectively to restore opposition using the flexor carpi ulnaris as a pulley and inserted into the APB.
- The Huber (abductor digiti quinti) transfer can effectively restore opposition and add thenar bulk. It is most often performed for congenital hypoplastic thumb cases.

The ability to oppose our thumbs has long been recognized as a defining characteristic of our humanity. Aristotle referred to this elegant and complex capability that we possess as one of the most distinctive human features. Bell[1] referred to opposition as "the distinguishing character of the human hand." By definition, opposition is the placement of the thumb in space in a position from which it can work. Sterling Bunnell[2] described this position of the thumb as "diametrically opposite the fingers with the thumb pulp facing the fingers and the thumb nail parallel to the volar surfaces of the fingers." It is important to distinguish the positional role of opposition (placement of the thumb opposite the long finger) from the power roles of grasp and pinch that occur following thumb opposition. This becomes particularly important when considering tendon transfers to restore opposition. Unlike the restoration of pinch, which requires powerful donor tendons, opposition transfers do not require large amounts of strength to achieve the goal of thumb positioning. The mechanics and vector of pull, however, are of paramount importance in restoring opposition.

## DEFINING OPPOSITION

In the simplest of terms, opposition is the placement of the thumb opposite the fingers. Maximal opposition occurs when the thumb is opposite the long finger. For contact with the index finger, less opposition is required. For contact with the ring and small fingers, the thumb will maximally oppose in line with the long finger. Simultaneously, the actions of the hypothenar musculature, in concert with the hypermobility of the fourth and fifth carpometacarpal (CMC) joints, allow for pulp-to-pulp contact between these ulnar digits and the thumb. One can appreciate this when attempting to achieve pulp-to-pulp contact between the thumb and all fingers in an alternating

OrthoCarolina, 1915 Randolph Road, Charlotte, NC 28211, USA
* Corresponding author.
*E-mail address:* glenn.gaston@orthocarolina.com

Hand Clin 32 (2016) 349–359
http://dx.doi.org/10.1016/j.hcl.2016.03.005
0749-0712/16/$ – see front matter © 2016 Elsevier Inc. All rights reserved.

fashion. Once fully opposed, tip-to-tip pinch between the thumb and all fingers requires very little movement of the thumb metacarpal. Almost all of the movement is by the fingers with small amounts of thumb metacarpophalangeal (MCP) and interphalangeal (IP) flexion.

The act of opposition requires 3 planar movements of the thumb metacarpal: palmar abduction, flexion, and pronation, all in a coordinated movement toward the pisiform. This "line of pull" makes the pisiform the ideal vector for restoring opposition. A beautifully orchestrated muscular balance is required for this unique motion to occur. The most influential muscles in opposition are the 3 intrinsic muscles of the thenar eminence: the abductor pollicis brevis (APB), the flexor pollicis brevis (FPB), and the opponens pollicis. Although its name would imply relevance, the abductor pollicis longus (APL) is somewhat of a misnomer. Although the APL often has some volar slips, also known as the digastric muscle of Wood, that contribute slightly to thumb palmar abduction, most of the slips insert onto the dorsum of the thumb metacarpal and contribute to thumb extension.[3–5] The APL is also a prime radial deviator of the wrist.

When one outlines the entire confluence of the thenar musculature, a triangular shape is apparent with an apex at the center of the volar base of the thumb proximal phalanx extending ulnarly at a nearly 90° angle toward the third metacarpal distally and scaphoid proximally. The distal margin of this triangle represents pure adduction (under greater control of the ulnar nerve) and the proximal margin pure palmar abduction (under greater control of the median nerve). The line bisecting the center represents the path of opposition and when followed leads directly toward the pisiform (**Fig. 1**).

## ANATOMY AND BIOMECHANICS

Understanding the anatomic position and physiologic function of the thumb intrinsic musculature allows a greater appreciation of the role of these 3 muscles in contributing to opposition. The most important muscle for opposition is the APB. It originates from the transverse metacarpal ligament as well as the tendon sheath of the flexor carpi radialis and the scaphotrapezium trapezoid joint capsule. The APB then runs along the radial border of the thumb metacarpal to insert into the abductor tubercle on the base of the proximal phalanx, thereby producing thumb metacarpophalangeal (MP) flexion and radial deviation, CMC joint flexion and palmar abduction, and IP extension through its contribution to the lateral bands (which

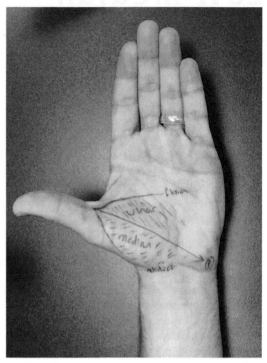

**Fig. 1.** Illustration of the thenar musculature triangle. The distal muscles contribute more to flexion and are under the control of the ulnar nerve predominately. The proximal muscles contribute more to palmar abduction and are under median nerve control. The line bisecting the triangle intersects the pisiform (P).

allows extension of IP to neutral in the absence of a functioning extensor pollicis longus [EPL]). When one considers that the APB has the lowest mass and tension fraction of any thenar muscle, anatomically speaking it is a small, weak muscle. Its unique anatomic position and mechanical advantage, however, make it the most influential muscle in thumb opposition. Being superficial to all other thenar muscles gives the APB the greatest mechanical advantage. This is enhanced dynamically, because when the deeper thenar muscles flex and shorten, the APB is forced further palmar, thus further increasing its mechanical advantage. It is for this reason that it is the most important muscle in opposition, despite the FPB having a larger cross-sectional diameter. An enthusiasm to restore "opposition strength" should be tempered with a recognition that opposition is a positional movement far more dependent on passive mobility and a proper line of pull than donor muscle power.

The FPB originates more medial (ulnar) off of the transverse carpal ligament than the APB and is often more distal as well. The FPB has 2 heads: a deep head more often innervated by the ulnar nerve and a superficial head more often innervated by the median nerve. Its deep head inserts onto the lateral sesamoid, which increases its lever distance for MP flexion, whereas the superficial head inserts into the abductor tubercle along with the APB. The FPB functions to flex and abduct the thumb metacarpophalangeal joint (MPJ), extend the IP joint (through its contributions to the lateral bands), and flex the CMC joint. Its more proximal fibers parallel the line of pull and function of the opponens pollicis (both median nerve innervated), and its more distal fibers parallel the function of the adductor pollicis (both ulnar nerve innervated). It is located in the center of the thenar triangle and not surprisingly has the most variability of its innervation of any thenar muscle. The relative contributions of the ulnar and median nerve to its function can have a significant impact on the amount of morbidity associated with an individual's median or ulnar nerve palsy.

The superficial head of the flexor pollicis brevis (FBP) is dually innervated by the median and ulnar nerve in approximately 30% of hands, and the deep head in 79%.[6,7] In a study assessing the effect of selective median nerve block at the wrist on thumb abduction, Boatright and Kiebzak[8] demonstrated that patients retained 30% of the abduction strength and with electromyographic correlation they noted superficial head of FBP paralysis in only 29% of patients. In the treatment of 147 patients with median nerve injuries over a 10-year period, Jensen[9] concluded that surgical restoration of opposition was indicated in only 14% of patients. In a recent study, Bertelli and colleagues[10] demonstrated that patients with an isolated high median nerve injury retained on average 7.5 out of 10.0 opposition function based on the Kapandji scale.[11]

The opponens pollicis originates from the transverse carpal ligament and the trapezium and inserts along the entire radial and dorsal ridge of the thumb metacarpal. It does not cross the MP joint and provides pronation as well as flexion and abduction of the CMC joint; it is the only thenar muscle that exerts no influence over the MP or IP joints. Because of its less important role in thumb opposition, Kaplan and others[12] have objected to the term opponensplasty, favoring instead "opposition tendon transfer."

The adductor pollicis is not truly a thenar muscle, as it does not reside in the thenar eminence (although some consider it and the first dorsal interosseous muscle thenar muscles as well). The adductor pollicis is the most important muscle in power pinch, although it is aided by the ulnar head of the FPB. All other thenar muscles in essence contribute to placing the thumb in the proper position so that the adductor and ulnar

head of the FPB can deliver pinch. It has the largest moment arm at the CMC joint of any muscle in the hand, giving it more importance than even the flexor pollicis longus in creating pinch power. The adductor pollicis inserts onto the medial sesamoid and ulnar base of the proximal phalanx and contributes to CMC and MP flexion, IP extension through the lateral bands, and supination of the thumb. The extensor pollicis longus also has a moment arm that produces adduction that in a normal hand contributes minimally to pinch; however, its role can become very important in the setting of a combined median and ulnar nerve palsy when it is the sole muscle remaining that can adduct the thumb and create pinch.

These 3 thenar muscles have an elegant interplay to position the thumb for work. The ensuing work may be either power pinch or more fine motor, and we have an amazing ability to uniquely position the thumb for either form of pinch that is required. There are 2 types of pinch: key pinch and tip pinch. Key pinch, also termed power grasp, requires a preparation phase performed by the APB and FPB intrinsic contributions to flex the MP joint and extend the IP joint. Then the adductor pollicis and deep head of the FPB fire to allow the thumb pulp to contact the lateral aspect of the index finger. In key pinch, the fingers simply must have sufficient MP flexion to receive the laterally directed force of the thumb and the thumb performs most of the work. Tip pinch and 3-point chuck pinch, also termed precision grasp, on the other hand, require much more digital control for this fine motor movement. The IP joint of the thumb is also positioned in slight flexion for precision grasp. The restoration of pinch and grasp is further discussed in the article (See Gaston RG, Cook S, Lourie GM: Ulnar Nerve Tendon Transfers for Pinch, in this issue).

## ETIOLOGY

There are many potential causes of median nerve palsy, and thus a lack of opposition. These include acute median nerve laceration or damage from trauma as well as chronic median nerve compression from carpal tunnel syndrome, pronator syndrome, or cervical radiculopathy. Also, congenital absence of thenar musculature is common with radial longitudinal deficiency and thumb hypoplasia. Many neurologic conditions, such as Charcot-Marie-Tooth, chronic inflammatory demyelinating polyneuropathy, and leprosy, frequently result in thenar muscle atrophy as well. Less common etiologies would include tumor or brachial plexopathies. In all cases of thenar muscle weakness, it is imperative to perform a meticulous sensory examination, as sensory loss can significantly impact the outcomes of tendon transfers.

## PHYSICAL EXAMINATION

The best way to assess APB atrophy is to view the thenar musculature from the radial side as opposed to from the traditional palmar side (ie, with the forearm in neutral rather than full supination). The strength of resisted palmar abduction is then tested and noted. It should be remembered that not all patients demonstrate a significant functional deficit in the presence of a median nerve palsy due to cross innervation or patient level of demand. The thumb MP joint should be assessed for hyperextension. The palmar plate of the thumb MP joint serves as a passive restraint to resist hyperextension forces. In a thumb with normal muscle balance, the intrinsic muscles of the thumb guard the joint against excessive load by serving as active restraints. In cases of muscle paralysis, however, the deprivation of the joint of its dynamic protection may result in gradual attenuation of the palmar plate with resultant MCP hyperextension.

Finally, in a low median nerve palsy, the thumb rests in constant unopposed external rotation and supination. Over time, in the absence of passive stretching exercises, this may result in progressive shortening and contracture of the dorsal first web space skin and fascia with resultant stiffness. If present, surgery to restore opposition must include elongation of the first webspace skin and fascia with either z-plasty or skin graft. Contracture of the first webspace will further place the MCP joint of the thumb at a biomechanical disadvantage and further predispose it to hyperextension deformity.

## SURGICAL PROCEDURES

As with all tendon transfer surgery, appropriate patient selection is paramount to an acceptable outcome. First and foremost, the patient must be clearly counseled about the nature of the surgery and the importance and general timeline of postoperative recovery and rehabilitation. Reasonable expectations for the outcome should be shared by the surgeon and patient, and the patient's willingness and ability to comply with postoperative instructions, including supervised hand therapy, should be ascertained. Soft tissue equilibrium should be achieved before considering tendon transfers.

To ensure an optimum setting for success, all articulations of the thumb should be supple to allow for effective excursion and effect of the transferred tendons. This often requires a period of regular and dedicated home exercises, supplemented by supervised hand therapy. Any adduction contracture must be corrected, and this can be assisted by a thermoplast first web "spacer" fashioned by the hand therapist. Available donors should be meticulously assessed, particularly in the setting of combined nerve injuries and relevant musculoskeletal trauma. For example, a combined median/ulnar nerve palsy, or multiple tendon lacerations of the wrist or forearm, may preclude the use of specific donors. The MCP joint of the thumb should be stable and significant laxity, particularly of the ulnar collateral ligament, can be addressed by joint arthrodesis.

### Extensor Indicis Proprius

Transfer of the extensor indicis proprius (EIP) to restore opposition offers several advantages, and is often the authors' preferred technique. It should be considered especially in the setting of previously lacerated flexor tendons (ie, a spaghetti wrist), and in the setting of a high median nerve palsy, in which most of the extrinsic digital flexors are not available donors. There is no risk of loss of grip strength (as with flexor digitorum superficialis [FDS] transfer), and it preserves the extrinsic digital flexors as donors for reconstruction of intrinsic function in combined median/ulnar nerve injuries. Finally, this does not require the surgical creation of a pulley, as the transfer around the ulna typically results in an ideal vector to achieve opposition.

A dorsal transverse incision is made just proximal to the MCP joint of the index finger, and the EIP is identified just ulnar and deep to the extensor digitorum communis to the index finger (**Fig. 2**A). The surgeon should be familiar with anatomic variations of the EIP at this level, including congenital absence, which has been observed in 0% to 4% of humans,[13] a radial position relative to extensor digitorum comminus (EDC) at the MCP joint 10% of the time, and multiple slips of EIP in 3% to 14% of cadaveric specimens.[14] The EIP is transected just proximal to the sagittal bands, as this typically yields just enough length to reach its target. Some investigators promote including additional length by harvesting an additional few centimeters of extensor hood[15,16]; however, we have found this to be unnecessary unless additional length is planned to be necessary for concurrent stabilization of the thumb MCP joint, such as in some congenital patients and combined median/ulnar nerve palsies. The distal stump of the EIP can then be sutured to the intact and more

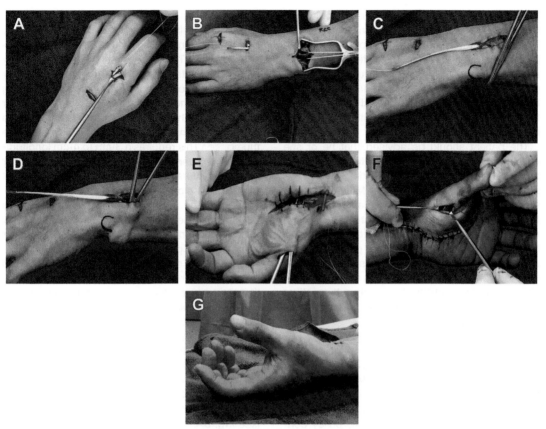

**Fig. 2.** EIP opponensplasty. (*A*) A dorsal transverse incision is made just proximal to the MCP joint of the index finger, and the EIP is identified just ulnar and deep to the EDC. It is transected just proximal to the sagittal bands. (*B, C*) Identification of the EIP musculotendinous junction through an incision made over fourth extensor compartment. Fascial attachments are divided and the EIP is pulled proximally into this incision. As in this patient, occasionally the EIP will not glide smoothly between these 2 incisions, and a counter incision over the dorsal-radial mid hand should be used to identify and divide any persistent fascial attachments. (*D*) A subcutaneous tunnel is developed around the ulna, and (*E*) also between the pisiform and the insertion site over the radial border of the thumb MCP. In the setting of a concurrent carpal tunnel release, as in this patient, an extensile carpal tunnel incision replaces the need for an incision just proximal to the pisiform. The EIP is passed subcutaneously around the ulna, into the carpal tunnel incision, then to the incision at the radial border of the thumb. (*F*) The tendon is sutured into place. (*G*) Appropriate tensioning results in the thumb resting palmarly abducted and opposite the index and middle fingers with the wrist at neutral.

radial EDC to allow for even distribution of pull across the MCP joint.

The next incision is made over the distal dorsal forearm at approximately the radial aspect of the ulnar neck, and the musculotendinous junction of the EIP is exposed. The EIP can be identified readily, as it has the most distal muscle belly of any muscle in the fourth compartment. Fascial attachments are divided and the EIP is pulled proximally into this incision. Occasionally the EIP will not glide smoothly between these 2 incisions, and a counter incision over the dorsal-radial mid hand should be used to identify and divide any persistent fascial attachments to neighboring structures (**Fig. 2**B, C). Another small incision is

made just proximal and ulnar to the pisiform, and the EIP is withdrawn through a subcutaneous tunnel created connecting this incision to the dorsal forearm incision. Care should be taken to avoid iatrogenic injury to the dorsal ulnar sensory branch. A final subcutaneous tunnel is then developed between the pisiform and the insertion site over the radial border of the thumb MCP (**Fig. 2**D). The ulna thus acts as the functional pulley for this tendon transfer, although some investigators advocate passing the EIP through a stab incision in the flexor carpi ulnaris.[17] In the setting of a concurrent carpal tunnel release, an extensile carpal tunnel incision obviates the need for the aforementioned incision just proximal to the pisiform: the

EIP can be passed subcutaneously around the ulna and into the carpal tunnel incision via one long tunnel (**Fig. 2**D, E). The EIP is passed, smooth gliding in the subcutaneous position is ensured, and the transferred tendon is sutured into place (**Fig. 2**F). Appropriate tensioning results in the thumb resting palmarly abducted and opposite the index and middle fingers with the wrist at neutral (**Fig. 2**G).

The patient should be advised that he or she may lose the ability to independently extend the index finger, and that there is theoretic risk of extension lag across the index finger MCP joint. In a series of patients with low median nerve palsy treated with EIP opponensplasty, Al-Qattan[17] noted 12 of 15 excellent results with no extension lag, and surmised that harvesting proximal to the extensor hood "eliminates" the risk of extension lag. Additionally, on rare occasion, there is insufficient length to reach the target, thus the patient should be consented for possible interpositional autograft, that is, palmaris longus.

### Flexor Digitorum Superficialis

The FDS of either the ring or middle finger is likely the most well described and widely used donor to achieve thumb opposition, with numerous variations in technique of donor harvest, pulley construction, and tendon insertion described. An absolute contraindication for this technique is high median nerve lesion, as all FDS musculature is devoid of innervation. Combined median/ulnar nerve lesions preclude the use of the ring finger FDS; however, the middle finger FDS can typically be used in this scenario, provided the middle finger flexor digitorum profundus (FDP) is not also ulnar nerve innervated only, which occurs in 5% of patients.[18]

The FDS is harvested through an incision typically overlying the A1 pulley of the ring (or middle) finger. Once the FDS is isolated, the finger is fully flexed, proximal traction on the FDS typically allows for visualization of the bifurcation of FDS at Campers chasm, and the FDS is transected at this level (**Fig. 3**A–C). Alternatively, a second incision can be made overlying the proximal interphalangeal joint (PIP) flexion crease of the finger, the A3 pulley can be divided, and FDS can be transected near its insertion into the middle phalanx. This more distal transection has potential drawbacks, including the risk of hyperextension of the PIP joint and subsequent development of swan neck deformity (especially in patients with preoperative hyperlaxity at the PIP joint), and also the risk of devascularizing the overlying FDP by disrupting the vincula at this level.[19]

Once the donor FDS has been harvested distally, there are 2 well-described options with regard to pulley formation and redirection to the thumb insertion site. The Thompson modification of the Royle FDS tendon transfer (the Thompson/Royle, or Royle/Thompson procedure) includes rerouting the FDS around the ulnar border of the palmar aponeurosis (the pulley) then subcutaneously to the thenar eminence and MCP joint of the thumb.[20,21] This requires a 3-cm to 4-cm longitudinal incision over the radial border of the hypothenar eminence, blunt dissection to the distal margin of the transverse carpal ligament, and careful identification of the ring finger FDS. Subcutaneous passage to the thumb MCP joint requires fairly aggressive blunt spreading, as the deep skin layer of the proximal palm is intimate with the palmar fascia. The vector of pull created with this technique is more suited to restore thumb flexion and abduction than true opposition, and thus this technique is more applicable in cases of combined median/ulnar nerve palsy in which there has been complete loss of intrinsic control of the thumb.

The other pulley option is the flexor carpi ulnaris (FCU) near its insertion into the pisiform, which yields a more effective line of pull to restore true thumb opposition. A several-centimeter incision is made over the most distal aspect of the FCU (see **Fig. 3**A, *dotted line*), the ringer finger FDS is identified and pulled proximally into this incision. In the setting of a concurrent carpal tunnel release, the FCU can be accessed through an extensile carpal tunnel incision (**Fig. 3**D). Attention is turned to fashioning the FCU into a pulley by passing the FDS through a simple midline slit or creation of a looped pulley with one-half of the FCU. A simple slit is created just proximal to the pisiform and it should be made long enough to allow for easy passage and glide of the FDS. A stay stitch should be placed at the proximal margin of the slit to prevent proximal propagation. A loop pulley is created by transecting the radial one-half of the split approximately 5 cm proximal to the pisiform, and suturing this radial slip to the intact ulnar half of the FCU distally (**Fig. 3**E, F). Great care should be taken while creating this pulley, as the ulnar neurovascular bundle lies in close proximity just radial to the FCU. The FDS is passed either directly through this loop or, preferably, around the ulnar intact half and then through the loop (see **Fig. 3**F).

Regardless of pulley technique, the tendon is then passed through a subcutaneous tunnel to the radial aspect of the thumb MCP, where a third incision is made and the FDS is either inserted into the ulnar base of the proximal phalanx or directly attached to the APB tendon (**Fig. 3**G). In patients who have developed instability of the

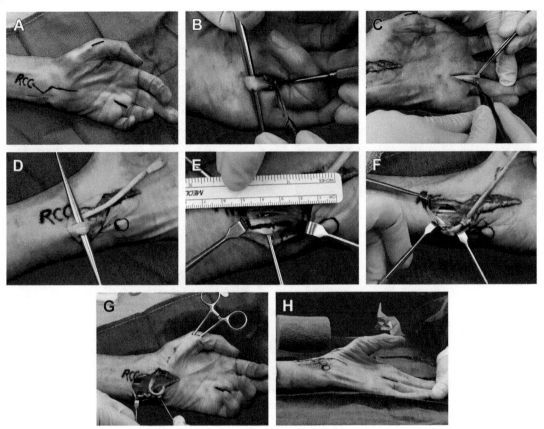

**Fig. 3.** FDP opponensplasty in an 87-year-old man with combined end-stage carpal tunnel syndrome, profound thenar atrophy, and ulnar neuropathy, absent palmaris, with intact ring finger FDS/FDP on preoperative examination. (*A*) The FDS is harvested through an incision over the ring finger A1 pulley. (*B, C*) Once the FDS is isolated, the finger is fully flexed, proximal traction on the FDS typically allows for visualization of the bifurcation of FDS at Camper chasm, and the FDS is transected. A several-centimeter incision can be made over the most distal aspect of the FCU (*A, dotted line*). (*D*) In this setting of a concurrent carpal tunnel release, both the proximal FDS and FCU can be accessed through an extensile carpal tunnel incision in lieu of a separate incision directly over the FCU. (*E, F*) A loop pulley is created in the FCU by transecting the radial one-half of a split approximately 5 cm proximal to the pisiform, and suturing this radial slip to the intact ulnar half of the FCU distally. The FDS is passed around the ulnar intact half and then through the loop. (*G*) The tendon is then passed through a subcutaneous tunnel to the radial aspect of the thumb MCP, where a third incision is made and the FDS is either inserted into the ulnar base of the proximal phalanx or directly attached to the APB tendon. (*H*) The transfer is tensioned such that passive wrist extension will result in full thumb opposition.

thumb MCP joint, and also in specific congenital cases (ie, lower-grade thumb hypoplasia), there is adequate length of transferred FDS to concurrently reconstruct the collateral ligaments. The transfer is tensioned such that passive wrist extension will result in full thumb opposition (**Fig. 3**H).

The ring finger FDS is the most commonly selected tendon for this transfer; however, the middle finger FDS also can be harvested in cases of high ulnar nerve palsy (harvesting FDS to ring finger would lead to the absence of extrinsic digital flexors). The patient should be counseled about potential loss of grip strength, particularly with use of the ring finger FDS.

## Palmaris Longus (Camitz)

A commonly used donor tendon to restore a component of opposition of the thumb is the palmaris longus (PL), and it is anatomically convenient when performing a carpal tunnel release in chronic cases. The PL can be harvested without any functional deficit, there is minimal donor site morbidity, and it functions synergistically with the APB. Before proceeding with this surgery, eponymized after Camitz,[22] it should be confirmed that the patient has a PL present, as congenital absence occurs in 15% to 20% of patients. If performing this procedure in concert with an open carpal tunnel release, the incision is

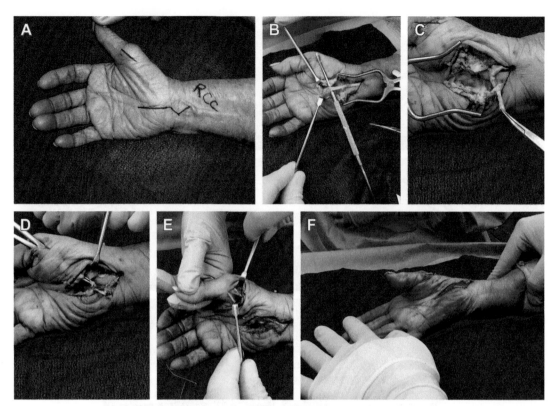

**Fig. 4.** PL opponensplasty (Camitz transfer) in an 81-year-old man with end-stage carpal tunnel syndrome and profound thenar atrophy. (*A*) An extensile carpal tunnel incision is made. (*B*) The PL is elongated with a 1.0-cm-wide to 1.5-cm-wide strip of palmar fascia. (*C–E*) A generous subcutaneous tunnel is then created between the distal forearm and the dorsoradial aspect of the thumb MCP joint, and an incision is made overlying the APB insertion, taking care to preserve the branch's radial sensory nerve. (*C*) The PL can be passed through a slit in the ulnar leaf of the release transverse carpal ligament to effect an appropriate pulley. (*E, F*) The fascial extension is then sutured to the APB tendon with the thumb placed in full passive abduction while the wrist is held neutral.

extended distally to approximately the distal palmar crease, and proximally in zig-zag fashion across the wrist flexion crease by several centimeters (**Fig. 4**A). The surgeon should be cognizant of the palmar cutaneous branch of the median nerve, which runs radial to the PL and in the radial floor of the flexor carpi radialis sheath, and can be avoided by directing the zig-zag ulnarly across the wrist. The PL is continuous distally with the pretendinous bands of the palmar aponeurosis, and to procure enough length to reach the thumb, the PL transfer is elongated with a 1.0-cm-wide to 1.5-cm-wide strip of this palmar fascia (**Fig. 4**B).

A generous subcutaneous tunnel is then created between the distal forearm and the dorsoradial aspect of the thumb MCP joint, and an incision is made overlying the APB insertion, taking care to preserve the branch's radial sensory nerve. The fascial extension is then sutured to the APB tendon with the thumb placed in full passive abduction while the wrist is held neutral (**Fig. 4**C–F).

It should be noted that this transfer has appropriately been referred to as an "abductorplasty" rather than an opponensplasty,[23] as the vector created only restores abduction and not pronation. This disadvantage may be overcome by passing the PL through a pulley created on the ulnar side of the flexor retinaculum[24] (see **Fig. 4**C), which results in a direction of pull from the pisiform to the thumb MCP joint. Subtle variations of modified Camitz procedures have been recently published, and good subjective and objective outcomes reported.[25–29]

There has been some debate about the necessity of performing a Camitz procedure concurrently with carpal tunnel release, as some investigators have reported gradual recovery of thenar atrophy after carpal tunnel release.[30,31] Conversely, insignificant improvement in thenar muscle function, despite recovery of sensory function, has been reported by others.[32,33] It seems reasonable to consider performing a concomitant Camitz procedure in cases of advanced carpal tunnel syndrome regardless of eventual thenar muscle recovery as, at a minimum, the transfer may act as a "placeholder" while incurring minimal added risk and morbidity to a carpal tunnel release.

## Abductor Digiti Minimi

Originally described by Huber,[34] transfer of the ulnar-nerve innervated abductor digit minimi (ADM) to restore opposition offers several advantages. The ADM is a predictably available donor in cases of isolated median nerve deficiency, and is especially applicable in patients with volar forearm or wrist trauma in which case other donors are either not available or would be able to glide effectively. Because of the similar dimension of the ADM to the APB, transfer of this muscle across the palm to the thumb also can help with cosmesis by restoring some of the bulk of the thenar eminence in cases of atrophy or congenital absence.

To harvest the ADM, an incision is designed extending from the ulnar base of the small finger to a point just proximal to the pisiform, thus exposing the entire broad muscle belly of ADM (**Fig. 5**A, B). The ADM insertion into the proximal phalanx and extensor mechanism is meticulously incised (**Fig. 5**C), maintaining as much length of the tendinous insertion as possible, and even including a small strip of periosteum if possible (especially applicable in children), ensuring

adequate length to reach the insertion site is paramount. The ADM is freed in a proximal direction and meticulously separated from the radially adjacent flexor digiti minimi. As dissection continues proximally, great care is taken to identify and preserve the major pedicle to the ADM, which emanates from the deep palmar branch of the ulnar artery and enters the muscle on its dorsal-radial border several millimeters distal to the pisiform.[35,36] The ADM originates from the pisiform, pisohamate ligament, and distal aspect of the FCU, and the more ulnar portions of this origin may need judicious release to achieve adequate excursion and rotation. A generous subcutaneous tunnel is created toward a second incision made over the APB insertion of the thumb (**Fig. 5**D), and the ADM is passed through the tunnel (**Fig. 5**E), requiring the surgeon to supinate the muscle 180°, similar to opening a page in a book. The thumb is placed in maximum opposition and the ADM is sutured appropriately. In rare cases, there is inadequate length, and augmentation with a free interpositional graft (ie, palmaris) is necessary.

## Others

A plethora of other tendon transfers to restore opposition have been described, and although used less frequently, these options are important for surgeons to keep in their arsenal for certain clinical scenarios. The extensor carpi ulnaris

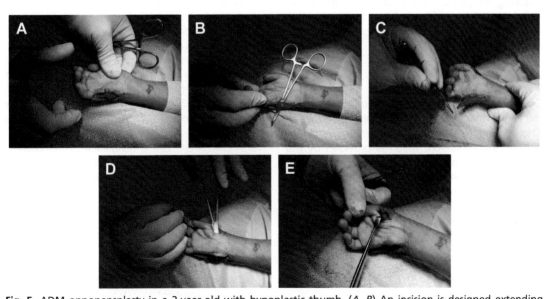

**Fig. 5.** ADM opponensplasty in a 2-year-old with hypoplastic thumb. (*A, B*) An incision is designed extending from the ulnar base of the small finger to a point just proximal to the pisiform, exposing the entire broad muscle belly of the ADM. (*C*) The ADM insertion into the proximal phalanx and extensor mechanism is incised. (*D*) A generous subcutaneous tunnel is created toward a second incision made over the APB insertion of the thumb, and (*E*) the ADM is passed through the tunnel.

(ECU)[37] can be released from its insertion on the fifth metacarpal and transferred to a recipient extensor pollicis brevis (EPB) tendon, which is released proximally at its musculotendinous junction and passed palmarly. Three incisions are required (dorsal thumb MP joint, dorsal ulnar wrist/forearm, and dorsal-radial forearm at EPB musculotendinous junction) and the ECU is passed subcutaneously from a point just proximal to the pisiform toward the thumb MCP joint to meet the EPB. The surgeon should ensure preoperatively that the patient has an intact FCU to prevent postoperative wrist imbalance and radial deviation. The extensor digit quinti proprius (EDQP) can be used with a similar path of transfer as the EIP; however, the surgeon must ensure there is an intact extensor digitorum communis to the small finger. Additionally, the donor tendon typically needs to be lengthened by including a strip of the extensor hood, and the patient must be counseled about the risk of extension lag at the small finger MCP joint.

Transfer of the radial wrist extensors (extensor carpi radialis brevis [ECRB] or extensor carpi radialis longus [ECRL]) has also been described,[38] rerouting the tendon around the ulnar aspect of the wrist in similar fashion to the EIP transfer, although to reach the APB insertion a free tendon interpositional graft is necessary. Alternatively, the ECRB or ECRL can be attached directly to a proximally transected recipient EPB or EPL.[39] Alternatively the brachioradialis can be used, again requiring interpositional graft, although Henderson found this to be less effective than the wrist extensors, but a useful option in the absence of other available donors.

## SUMMARY

Opposition is the placement of the thumb opposite the fingers into a position from which it can work. This motion requires thumb palmar abduction, flexion, and pronation, which is provided by the APB, FPB, and opponens pollicis. In the setting of a median nerve palsy, this function is typically lost, although anatomic variations and the dual innervation of the FPB may prevent complete loss at times. There are multiple well-described and accepted tendon transfers to restore opposition, none of which have been proven to be superior to the others.

## REFERENCES

1. Bell C. The hand: its mechanism and vital endowments as evincing designs. 3rd edition. London: William Pickering; 1834.

2. Bunnell S. Opposition of the thumb. J Bone Joint Surg 1938;20:269–84.

3. Khoury Z, Bertelli J, Gilbert A. The subtendons of the abductor pollicislongus muscle. Surg Radiol Anat 1991;13(3):245e246.

4. El-Beshbishy RA, Abdel-Hamid GA. Variations of the abductor pollicislongus tendon: an anatomic study. Folia Morphol (Warsz) 2013; 72(2):161e166.

5. Roh MS, Strauch RJ, Xu L, et al. Thenar insertion of abductor pollicislongus accessory tendons and thumb carpometacarpal osteoarthritis. J Hand Surg Am 2000;25(3):458–63.

6. Zancolli EA, Ziadenberg C, Zancolli E. Biomechanics of the trapeziometacarpal joint. Clin Orthop Relat Res 1987;220:14–26.

7. Olave E, Prates JC, Del Sol M, et al. Distribution patterns of the muscular branch of the median nerve in the thenar region. J Anat 1995; 186(Pt 2):441–6.

8. Boatright JR, Kiebzak GM. The effects of low median nerve block on thumb abduction strength. J Hand Surg Am 1997;22(5):849–52.

9. Jensen EG. Restoration of opposition of the thumb. Hand 1978;10(2):161–7.

10. Bertelli JA, Soldado F, Lehn VL, et al. Reappraisal of clinical deficits following high median nerve injuries. J Hand Surg Am 2016;41(1):13–9.

11. Kapandji A. Clinical test of apposition and counterapposition of the thumb. Ann Chir Main 1986;5(1): 67e73.

12. Posner MA, Kapila D. Restoration of opposition. Hand Clin 2012;28:27–44.

13. Trivedi S, Siddiqui AU, Sinha TP, et al. Absence of extensor indices; a rare anatomical variant. Int J Biol Res 2014;05(01):61–2.

14. Gonzalez MH, Weinzweig N, Kay T, et al. Anatomy of the extensor tendons to the index finger. J Hand Surg 1996;21A:988–99.

15. Burkhalter W, Christensen RC, Brown P. Extensor indicis proprius opponensplasty. J Bone Joint Surg Am 1973;55:725–32.

16. Anderson GA, Lee V, Sundararaj GD. Opponensplasty by extensor indicis and flexor digitorum superficialis tendon transfer. J Hand Surg Br 1992; 17:611–4.

17. Al-Qattan MH. Extensor indicis proprius opponensplasty for isolated traumatic low median nerve palsy: a case series. Can J Plast Surg 2012; 20(4):255–7.

18. Bhadra N, Keith MW, Peckham PH. Variations in innervation of the flexor digitorum profundus muscle. J Hand Surg 1999;24:700–3.

19. North ER, Littler JW. Transferring the flexor superficialis tendon. Technical considerations in the prevention of proximal interphalangeal joint disability. J Hand Surg 1980;5:498–501.

20. Royle ND. An operation for paralysis of the intrinsic muscles of the thumb. JAMA 1938;111: 612–3.

21. Thompson TC. A modified operation for opponens paralysis. J Bone Joint Surg 1942;24:632–40.

22. Camitz H. Surgical treatment of paralysis of opponens muscle of thumbs. Acta Chir Scand 1929;65: 77–81.

23. Smith RJ. Tendon transfers of the hand and forearm. Boston: Little Brown; 1987. p. 57–83.

24. MacDougal BA. Palmaris longus opponensplasty. Plast Reconstr Surg 1995;96(4):982–4.

25. Park IJ, Kim HM, Lee SU, et al. Opponensplasty using palmaris longus tendon and flexor retinaculum pulley in patients with severe carpal tunnel syndrome. Acta Orthop Trauma Surg 2010;130(7): 829–34.

26. Kang SW, Chung YG, Lee JY, et al. Modified Camitz opponensplasty using transverse carpal ligament loop pulley in patients with advanced carpal tunnel syndrome. Plast Reconstr Surg 2012;129(4):761–3.

27. Naeem R, Lahiri A. Modified Camitz opponensplasty for severe thenar wasting secondary to carpal tunnel syndrome: case series. J Hand Surg Am 2013;38(4): 795–8.

28. Kato N, Yoshizawa T, Sakai H. Simultaneous modified Camitz opponensplasty using a pulley at the radial side of the flexor retinaculum in severe carpal tunnel syndrome. J Hand Surg Eur Vol 2013;39(6): 632–6.

29. Hattori Y, Doi K, Sakamoto S, et al. Camitz tendon transfer using flexor retinaculum as a pulley in advanced carpal tunnel syndrome. J Hand Surg Am 2014;39(12):2454–9.

30. Mondelli M, Reale F, Padua R, et al. Clinical and neurophysiological outcome of surgery in extreme carpal tunnel syndrome. Clin Neurophysiol 2001; 112(7):1237–42.

31. Park IJ, Kim BJ. Prognosis of carpal tunnel release with extreme thenar atrophy. J Korean Soc Surg Hand 2002;7:52–6.

32. Littler JW, Li CS. Primary restoration of thumb opposition with median nerve decompression. Plast Reconstr Surg 1967;39(1):74–5.

33. Foucher G, Malizos C, Sammut D, et al. Primary palmaris longus transfer as an opponensplasty in carpal tunnel release. A series of 73 cases. J Hand Surg Eur Vol 1991;16(1):56–60.

34. Huber E. Hilfsoperation bet median uhlahmung. Dtsch Arch Klin Med 1921;136:271 [in German].

35. Dunlap J, Manske PR, McCarthy JA. Perfusion of the abductor digitiquinti after transfer on a neurovascular pedicle. J Hand Surg Am 1989;14:992–5.

36. Uysal AC, Alagöz MS, Tüccar E, et al. The vascular anatomy of the abductor digitiminimi and the flexor digitiminimi brevis muscles. J Hand Surg 2005; 30A:172–6.

37. Phalen GS, Miller RC. The transfer of wrist extensor muscles to restore or reinforce flexion of power of the fingers and opposition the thumb. J Bone Joint Surg 1947;29:993–7.

38. Henderson ED. Transfer of wrist extensors and brachioradialis to restore opposition of the thumb. J Bone Joint Surg 1962;44:513–22.

39. Kaplan I, Dinner M, Chait L. Use of extensor pollicislongus tendon as a distal extension for an opposition transfer. Plast Reconstr Surg 1976;57: 186–90.

# A Comprehensive Guide on Restoring Grasp Using Tendon Transfer Procedures for Ulnar Nerve Palsy

 CrossMark

Rafael J. Diaz-Garcia, MD[a,b,*], Kevin C. Chung, MD, MS[c]

## KEYWORDS

• Ulnar • Nerve • Tendon • Transfer • Grasp

## KEY POINTS

• Loss of ulnar nerve function causes significant disability to the upper extremity because of loss of function of the intrinsic muscles of the hand.
• Ulnar nerve paralysis results in weakened and uncoordinated grasp caused by loss of the principal flexors of the metacarpophalangeal joint.
• Dynamic transfers for restoration of grasp tend to have better surgical outcomes, but they may not be available in patients with combined nerve palsy.
• Correction of deformity and digital posture is more predictable than improvement of strength with tendon transfers.

## INTRODUCTION

The versatility, finesse, and strength of the human hand depend on the delicate interplay between the intrinsic and extrinsic muscles.[1] Loss of ulnar nerve function causes a complex and multidimensional disability in the hand; what results is deformed, weakened, and uncoordinated. Most commonly, the cause is trauma to the brachial plexus or the ulnar nerve; other causes include leprosy, poliomyelitis, and Charcot-Marie-Tooth disease.[2] To address this difficult problem, surgeons must have a thorough understanding of the anatomy and function, as well as the reconstructive goals, of the patient. Tendon transfers take advantage of muscular and mechanical redundancy to improve functional performance by redistribution of available assets.[3] This article reviews the biomechanics of grasp and the deficits that result from ulnar nerve paralysis. It also discusses how to improve function by the restoration of balance in the digits via tendon transfer.

### Biomechanics of Grasp

Initiating grasp of an object requires a coordinated effort between the intrinsic and extrinsic tendons of the hand. Flexion of the proximal phalanx at the metacarpophalangeal (MCP) joint is chiefly accomplished by the ulnar nerve–innervated

Disclosures: The authors have no financial disclosures or conflicts of interest to disclose related to this work. K.C. Chung was supported by the National Institute of Arthritis and Musculoskeletal and Skin Diseases of the National Institutes of Health under award number 2 K24-AR053120-06. The content is solely the responsibility of the authors and does not necessarily represent the official views of the National Institutes of Health.
<sup>a</sup> Division of Plastic Surgery, Department of Surgery, Allegheny General Hospital, Allegheny Health Network, 320 East North Avenue, Suite 401, Pittsburgh, PA 15212, USA; <sup>b</sup> University of Pittsburgh School of Medicine, Pittsburgh, PA 15260, USA; <sup>c</sup> Section of Plastic Surgery, Department of Surgery, University of Michigan, Ann Arbor, MI 48109, USA
* Corresponding author. Division of Plastic Surgery, Allegheny General Hospital, 320 East North Avenue, Suite 401, Pittsburgh, PA 15212.
E-mail address: rjdiazgarcia@gmail.com

interossei. The interossei tendons cross the MCP joints volar to the axis of rotation to insert on the lateral bands of the dorsal extensor mechanism. Because of this anatomy, muscular contraction can both flex the MCP and extend the interphalangeal (IP) joints. In normal digital flexion, there is synchrony of the MCP and IP joints, so that closure of a fist is fluid in motion. MCP flexion is driven by intrinsic activation, and the extrinsic flexors power IP flexion. The lumbricals also assist in flexion of the MCP joint, but their main function is in the extension of the IP joints, often referred to as the workhorse of the extensor mechanism.[4] The lumbrical muscles are intriguing and elegant structures that originate from the flexor digitorum profundus tendons and insert into the lateral bands of the extensor mechanism; their main function is to modulate the flexor and extensor mechanisms for smooth movement of the fingers.[5] Termination of grasp and digital extension involve the interplay of the intrinsic muscles with the extrinsic extensors. MCP extension is obtained through the sagittal bands, and, as long as hyperextension does not occur at that joint, there is sufficient excursion in the extrinsic extensor tendon to result in interphalangeal extension as well.

### Pathophysiology of Deficit

With classic low ulnar nerve paralysis, there is complete loss of function of the interossei and the 2 ulnar lumbricals, resulting in a loss of the primary flexors of the MCP joints and extensors of the IP joints. The extrinsic flexors can compensate for this loss, but the flexor digitorum superficialis (FDS) and flexor digitorum profundus (FDP) tendons only flex the MCP once the IP joints have reached maximum flexion. This condition causes asynchronous flexion of the digit and the characteristic roll-up flexion of the ulnar claw hand.[6] It can be difficult for patients with ulnar nerve paralysis to grasp larger objects, because the flexed fingertips often push the object out of the grasp (**Fig. 1**).

Clawing develops because the loss of tone in the intrinsic muscles causes the MCP joints to hyperextend and the sagittal bands to be parallel to the course of the tendon.[4] The extensor tendon thus exerts all of its force on the proximal phalanx and remains lax more distally. The normal elastic properties of the extrinsic flexors result in the IP joints flexing when the MCP hyperextends. Supple joints are a prerequisite to success with any tendon transfer. The Bouvier test is performed to differentiate between those patients who only need improvement of MCP joint flexion and those who require augmentation of IP extension (**Table 1**). To perform it, the MCP joints are blocked from extension and the patient is asked to actively extend the IP joints. A positive test shows good IP extension and implies central slip competency and that addressing the MCP hyperextension deformity alone will improve digital function. These patients are thought to have a simple claw hand. A static procedure, such as MCP capsulodesis or arthrodesis, provides a biomechanical advantage for the extensor tendons to extend the IP joints adequately, although it fails to add any additional power to the grasp. A negative Bouvier reflects incompetence of the extensor mechanism and is referred to as a complex claw hand for the sake of this discussion. This patient population requires a transfer that not only improves MCP posture but also augments extension.

Not only does the paralysis of the intrinsic musculature cause awkward and poorly coordinated digital motion but it greatly reduces grip strength in the affected hand. Loss of grip strength has been estimated to be between 50% and 75%, and is multifactorial.[4,7] The median nerve–innervated lumbricals mitigate the clawing in the index and middle fingers, but grip strength in these digits is also weak in flexion/grasp. High ulnar nerve paralysis adds the loss of the ulnar half of the FDP, which further weakens grip strength and grasp.

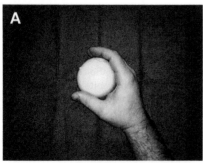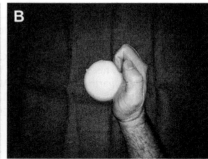

**Fig. 1.** (*A*) Normal synchronous flexion for attempted grasp of a large object versus (*B*) abnormal roll-up flexion for attempted grasp of a large object. Note the lack of MCP flexion in the latter until maximum IP joint flexion.

| Table 1 Reconstructive options for grasp in the hand with ulnar paralysis | | |
|---|---|---|
| **Bouvier Test** | **Operation** | **Benefits/Limitations** |
| Positive: simple claw | Zancolli capsulodesis | Easy to complete and minimal morbidity. Likely to stretch over time. Should only be used in combined nerve palsies because of lack of donors |
| | FDS lasso | Fairly easy to complete. May provide increase in grip strength. May result in swan-neck deformity caused by loss of FDS at PIP |
| Negative: complex claw | FDS 4-tail transfer | Greatest correction of claw deformity, particularly in patients with long-standing paralysis. Technically challenging. May result in swan-neck deformity caused by loss of FDS at PIP. Our preferred option, unless contraindicated |
| | ECRL/ECRB 4-tail transfer | Technically challenging. May be prone to scarring caused by passing through intermetacarpal space to recreate intrinsic function from dorsum of wrist. Requires tendon grafts. Our second option, if FDS to long finger is unavailable |

*Abbreviations:* FDS, flexor digitorum superficialis; PIP, proximal interphalangeal.

## SURGICAL TECHNIQUE
### Simple Claw Hand Reconstructions

Static reconstructions address the ulnar claw deformity by preventing MCP hyperextension and allowing the extrinsic extensors to extend the IP joints. In addition, they assist in grasp by placing the MCP joint in some degree of flexion. Numerous approaches have been described, including the use of dorsal bone blocks at the MCP joint,[8] capsular plication/advancement,[9–11] release of the A1/A2 pulleys,[12] and tenodesis.[13,14] One choice is MCP capsulodesis by volar plate advancement with the use of bone anchors, although dynamic reconstruction is always preferable. However, with any soft tissue–type procedure, stretching out of the soft tissue construct is common and loss of MCP joint flexion is foreseeable. The most predictable procedure for maintenance of MCP joint flexion is arthrodesis. MCP arthrodesis is particularly useful in combined high median and ulnar nerve injuries, in which there is a lack of dynamic tendon transfer options.

The potential efficacy of the static procedures must be tested preoperatively with the Bouvier maneuver (discussed earlier) to ensure sufficient IP extension from the extrinsic tendons.

- They do not improve flexion synchrony or increase grip strength.
- They are the only choice in the setting of combined nerve injuries with a paucity of donor motors for tendon transfers.

### Metacarpophalangeal Capsulodesis

A 3-cm to 4-cm incision is made over the A1 pulleys of the ring and small fingers, in line with the distal palmar crease. Protecting the neurovascular bundles, the A1 pulleys are exposed and released longitudinally, allowing exposure of the volar plate of the MCP joint. A distally based, rectangular-shaped flap of volar plate is created by releasing the proximal attachment from the metacarpal and creating 2 longitudinal incisions. A bone anchor is placed or a bone tunnel is created at the metacarpal neck to establish proximal advancement of the volar plate to create at least a 30° flexion contracture. Sutures are cinched down, the incision is closed with nylon, and the patient is placed in a dorsal blocking splint with the MCPs flexed.

### Flexor Digitorum Superficialis Lasso

A 3-cm to 4-cm incision is made over the A1 pulleys of the ring and small fingers, in line with the distal palmar crease (**Fig. 2**). The neurovascular bundles are protected, and the A1 and A2 pulleys are exposed. In high ulnar nerve injuries, a separate Bruner incision is made over the palmar aspect of the middle finger for FDS harvest. A transverse slit is made at the A3 pulley to release the FDS tendon at the level of the A2 pulley to preserve the FDS insertion to prevent hyperextension deformity of the proximal interphalangeal (PIP) joint from the loss of FDS attachment. The FDS tendon is retrieved under the A2 and sutured back to itself, so as to create a tendinous loop around the A1 pulley (**Fig. 3**). The FDS tensioning is done with the wrist in neutral position so as to set the ring and small finger MCP joints in flexion and recreate the normal resting cascade from index to small. The incisions are closed with nylon and the patient is placed in a dorsal splint with the MCPs flexed.

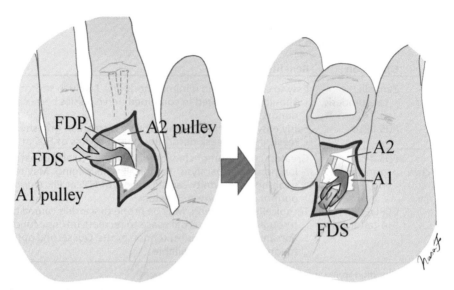

**Fig. 2.** FDS lasso procedure. A loop is created at the A1 pulley with the FDS tendon to create a flexion contracture at the MCP joint.

## Complex Claw Hand Reconstructions

Dynamic reconstruction after ulnar nerve palsy transfer uses an active motor unit to correct the MCP hyperextension deformity that results in the characteristic clawing. They have the added benefits of potentially improving IP joint extension and improving grip strength, depending on the tendinous insertion site on transfer. Digital flexors can serve as local donor sites with good tendinous length, but grip strength is more predictably improved with wrist extensors or flexors. However, wrist tendons such as the ECRB cannot reach the lateral bands; therefore, tendon grafts are often used, which can have problems with tendon adhesions and rupture. Alternatively, the ECRB can be z-lengthened after releasing its insertion and flipped distally on itself to double its length. It can then be divided into 2 tails for transfer. The FDS option, if available, is our preferred option. Also, the need for other tendon transfers that accompany ulnar nerve palsy, such as the restoration of pinch, must be considered. Often, a dorsal

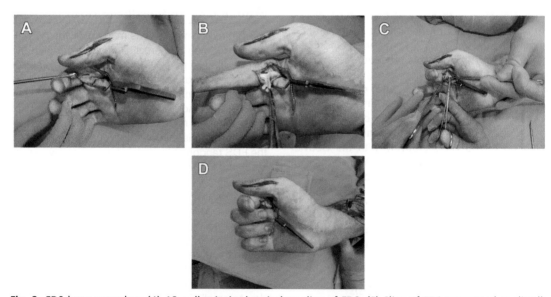

**Fig. 3.** FDS lasso procedure (*A*) A3 pulley incised to isolate slips of FDS. (*B*) Slips of FDS transected as distally as possible. (*C*) Slips of FDS folded proximally to create flexion at MCP joint. (*D*) Improved posture of digit after suture of FDS back onto itself.

donor is considered for one (ECRB) and a palmar donor (FDS) for the other function. This possibility must be considered in the preoperative planning for restoring both pinch and grasp.

- Dynamic transfers can improve flexion synchrony and improve grip strength.
- Dynamic transfers can improve IP joint extension if inserted into the lateral bands; this is required if negative Bouvier maneuver. If transfers are placed into the lateral bands for a Bouvier-positive maneuver a swan-neck deformity may occur, especially in ligamentously lax individuals.
- Dynamic transfers can be inserted into the base of the proximal phalanx if the Bouvier maneuver is positive.

### Stiles-Bunnell Flexor Digitorum Superficialis Transfer

A Bruner incision is planned and incised over the PIP joints of the affected digits. A separate incision is made over the proximal phalanx between the glabrous and nonglabrous skin to expose the radial lateral band (**Fig. 4**). Similar to the Zancolli lasso, the FDS of the middle finger is used as a donor in the setting of high ulnar nerve injuries because this tendon is innervated by the intact median nerve. The A3 pulley is opened and the FDS is divided as distally as possible, with the chiasm split into 2 slips as proximally as possible. The FDS is passed through the lumbrical canal with a tendon passer or hemostat to reach the radial aspect of the small

and ring fingers, deep to the radial neurovascular bundles. It is key to remain palmar to the deep transverse metacarpal ligament while passing the slips of FDS, so that the force remains palmar to the axis of rotation at the MCP joint. The slips are then tensioned through the radial lateral band with the wrist at neutral, once again trying to recreate the digital cascade and MP flexion of 70° or greater (**Fig. 5**). Passive wrist flexion should result in full MP extension with appropriate tension. Incisions are closed with nylon and the patient is placed in an intrinsic-plus splint.

### Wrist Extensor-to-Intrinsic Transfer

The Brand intrinsic transfer classically uses the extensor carpi radialis brevis (ECRB) as the motor unit to power the improvement of grip strength and restoration of IP extension[15] (**Fig. 6**). However, ECRB is our preferred transfer for restoration of pinch, so extensor carpi radialis longus (ECRL)[16,17] or FCR[13] can be used instead. If a dynamic option is selected and the FDS tendon is not an available donor (ie, in the setting of ulnar nerve injury in combination with high median nerve injury), then the ECRL or ECRB option is most suitable. A transverse or oblique incision is made over the distal aspect of the second compartment, near the tendinous insertion on the metacarpal base of choice. Small transverse incisions are made over the metacarpal necks in the interspace of the second and third metacarpals and fourth and fifth metacarpals. Tendon grafts are harvested from the donor site of choice, be it

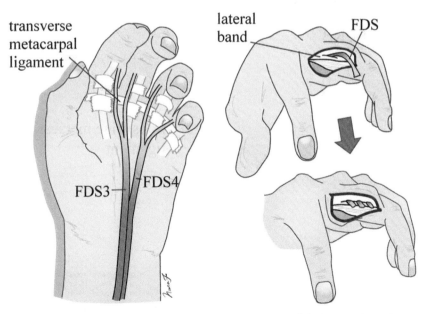

**Fig. 4.** Stiles-Bunnell FDS 4-tail transfer. In low ulnar nerve palsy, the FDS of the long and ring fingers can be transferred to the lateral bands of all the digits to improve digital posture and coordination in flexion and extension.

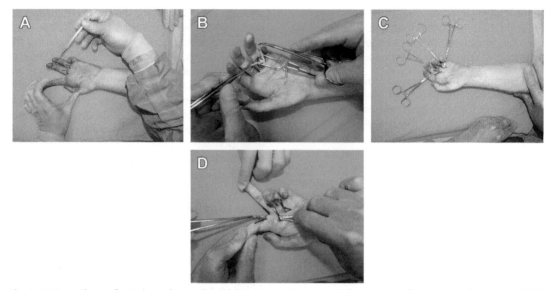

**Fig. 5.** FDS 4-tail transfer in low ulnar palsy (*A*) Bruner incision on middle and ring fingers to isolate slips of FDS. (*B*) Slips of FDS transected as distally as possible. (*C*) Slips of FDS separated from one another proximally. (*D*) Slips of FDS transferred through lumbrical canal to the lateral bands of the dorsal extensor hood and tensioned with the wrist in neutral.

palmaris, plantaris, or the long toe extensors, with a total of 4 tails created. From this dorsal incision, they are passed volar to the deep intermetacarpal ligament and into dorsal digital incisions. The grafts are firmly fixed to the radial lateral band of the middle through small finger and the ulnar lateral band of the index. Once an open and unimpeded path is confirmed for the each of the grafts, they are sutured to the wrist extensor. Appropriate tension is obtained with maximal wrist extension and the digits

in the intrinsic-plus position and confirmed with MP extension on wrist flexion. Incisions are closed with nylon and the patient is placed in an intrinsic-plus splint.

## Flexor Digitorum Profundus Side-to-Side Transfer for High Ulnar Nerve

In high ulnar nerve injuries, there is an additional loss of the ulnar half of the FDP with loss of distal

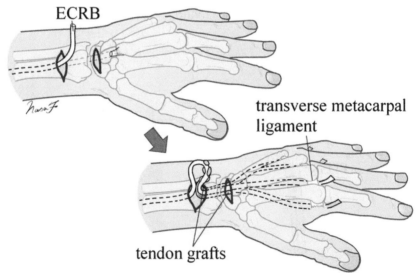

**Fig. 6.** Brand 4-tail transfer. A wrist extensor, such as the ECRB, can be transferred with the aid of tendon grafts to the lateral bands of each digit to recreate intrinsic function. The tendon grafts must pass through the interossei and below the transverse metacarpal ligament, predisposing them to adhesions.

interphalangeal (DIP) flexion in the ring and small fingers. This loss is addressed with a side-to-side transfer at the wrist, uniting the small and ring finger FDP tendons to the median nerve–innervated middle finger FDP tendon. The index FDP is left undisturbed, because independent flexion of this digit is important.

## REHABILITATION AND RECOVERY

Customarily, after all of these procedures, the patient is splinted with the MCP joints in 60° to 70° of flexion and with the IP joints in full extension until the first postoperative visit. If the lateral bands were not a part of the reconstructive procedure, the IP joints can be left free to do gentle range-of-motion exercises. After the first postoperative visit, the patient is kept in an intrinsic-plus orthosis for an additional 2 to 4 weeks, before commencing active range-of-motion exercises in a dorsal blocking splint. An additional 4 weeks of reeducation are needed before releasing the patient to all activities. All orthotics are discontinued at 2 months postoperatively, but therapy may continue for several weeks.

More recently, hand surgeons have extrapolated knowledge about flexor tendon repairs and have been advocating for early active motion after tendon transfers for ulnar claw deformity. A prospective trial of immediate postoperative active mobilization after FDS 4-tail transfer saw no incidence of tendon rupture and no clinically relevant difference in correction of claw deformity in patients with leprosy compared with historical controls.[18] However, recovery was on average 3 weeks faster and pain relief was better in those who began immediate mobilization protocols. This finding was confirmed in a subsequent randomized control trial.[19]

## CLINICAL RESULTS IN THE LITERATURE

There are multiple reconstructive options for the restoration of grasp after ulnar nerve paralysis for 2 key reasons. First and foremost, the patient population is heterogeneous and the reconstructive plan needs to be customized to the patient's goals, deficits, and available motors to transfer. This requirement is most apparent with combined nerve injuries, for which priorities have to be made and static grasp reconstructions may be preferred to preserve a motor for another reconstruction. The second reason is that there is no perfect reconstruction, and thus tradeoffs must be accepted. Static reconstructions, such as volar plate advancement, are a simpler option that can be used for patients with a positive Bouvier

test or with combined neuropathies. Brown[10] published a series of 44 patients treated with capsulodesis and concluded that less than 50% of the hands were improved with regard to clawing, more efficient grasp, and/or increased strength.

The Zancolli lasso procedure and FDS 4-tail transfer can provide a dynamic reconstruction to improve MCP flexion, and some proponents claim that grip strength is increased. Ozkan and colleagues[20] evaluated their results comparing the efficacy of FDS transfer, ECRL transfer, and Zancolli lasso in 44 patients with irreparable ulnar nerve injuries and with a mean follow-up of greater than or equal to 3 years. ECRL transfer and Zancolli lasso restored grip strength most effectively, and they were most efficacious in patients with short-standing paralysis. This improvement in strength is related to improved digital posture, as opposed to greater force in flexion. FDS transfer was most efficacious in addressing the claw deformity, particularly in patients with long-standing paralysis. All groups saw a mild improvement in grip strength from their preoperative state, ranging from 7% to 15%. However, most studies have shown that grip strength is affected minimally and may be decreased when using the FDS for intrinsic reconstruction.[21] Harvest of FDS may result in swan-neck deformity caused by the unchecked force of the central slip on the middle phalanx. Swan-neck deformity was seen in 1 digit in numerous patients, with those numbers ranging from 15% to almost 85% of patients who underwent FDS transfer for grasp.[20,22,23]

## SUMMARY

Ulnar nerve paralysis presents the greatest challenge for functional recovery for hand surgeons performing tendon transfers. Correction of the deformity can be done predictably with practice, but true restoration of function is all but impossible. Grip strength is difficult to recreate and complications can result, be they swan-neck deformities or significant postoperative adhesions of the transfers. Surgical planning based on patient need, hand deficit, and available tendons helps to provide tailored reconstructive strategies for each patient.

## ACKNOWLEDGMENTS

The authors thank Nasa Fujihara for her skillful artwork in this article.

## REFERENCES

1. Chase R. Muscle tendon kinetics. Am J Surg 1965;
109:277–82.

2. Riordan DC. Tendon transfers for nerve paralysis of the hand and wrist. Curr Pract Orthop Surg 1964; 23:17–40.

3. Omer GE. Tendon transfers for traumatic nerve injuries. J Hand Surg 2004;4(3):214–26.

4. Smith RJ. Tendon transfers of the hand and forearm. 1st edition. Boston: Little, Brown; 1987.

5. Wang K, McGlinn EP, Chung KC. A biomechanical and evolutionary perspective on the function of the lumbrical muscle. J Hand Surg 2014;39(1):149–55.

6. Srinivasan H. Clinical features of paralytic claw fingers. J Bone Joint Surg 1979;61(7):1060–3.

7. Goldfarb CA, Stern PJ. Low ulnar nerve palsy. J Am Soc Surg Hand 2003;3(1):14–26.

8. Mikhail IK. Bone block operation for clawhand. Surg Gynecol Obstet 1964;118:1077–9.

9. Zancolli EA. Claw-hand caused by paralysis of the intrinsic muscles: a simple surgical procedure for its correction. J Bone Joint Surg 1957;39-A(5): 1076–80.

10. Brown PW. Zancolli capsulorrhaphy for ulnar claw hand. Appraisal of forty-four cases. J Bone Joint Surg 1970;52(5):868–77.

11. Srinivasan H. Dermadesis and flexor pulley advancement: first report on a simple operation for correction of paralytic claw fingers in patients with leprosy. J Hand Surg 1985;10(6 Pt 2):979–82.

12. Bunnell S. Surgery of the intrinsic muscles of the hand other than those producing opposition of the thumb. J Bone Joint Surg 1942;24(1):1–31.

13. Riordan DC. Tendon transplantations in median-nerve and ulnar-nerve paralysis. J Bone Joint Surg 1953;35-A(2):312–20. passim.

14. Parkes A. Paralytic claw fingers–a graft tenodesis operation. Hand 1973;5(3):192–9.

15. Brand P. Tendon grafting. Illustrated by a new operation for intrinsic paralysis of the fingers. J Bone Joint Surg Br 1961;43:444–53.

16. Burkhalter WE. Restoration of power grip in ulnar nerve paralysis. Orthop Clin North Am 1974;5(2): 289–303.

17. Burkhalter WE, Strait JL. Metacarpophalangeal flexor replacement for intrinsic muscle paralysis. J Bone Joint Surg 1973;55A:1656–76.

18. Rath S. Immediate postoperative active mobilization versus immobilization following tendon transfer for claw deformity correction in the hand. J Hand Surg 2008;33(2):232–40.

19. Rath S, Selles RW, Schreuders TA, et al. A randomized clinical trial comparing immediate active motion with immobilization after tendon transfer for claw deformity. J Hand Surg 2009; 34(3):488–94, 494.e1–5.

20. Ozkan T, Ozer K, Gulgonen A. Three tendon transfer methods in reconstruction of ulnar nerve palsy. J Hand Surg 2003;28(1):35–43.

21. Hastings H 2nd, McCollam SM. Flexor digitorum superficialis lasso tendon transfer in isolated ulnar nerve palsy: a functional evaluation. J Hand Surg 1994;19(2):275–80.

22. Brandsma JW, Ottenhoff-De Jonge MW. Flexor digitorum superficialis tendon transfer for intrinsic replacement. Long-term results and the effect on donor fingers. J Hand Surg 1992;17(6):625–8.

23. Reddy NR, Kolumban SL. Effects of fingers of leprosy patients having surgical removal of sublimus tendons. Lepr India 1981;53(4):594–9.

# Ulnar Nerve Tendon Transfers for Pinch

Shane Cook, MD[a],*, R. Glenn Gaston, MD[b], Gary M. Lourie, MD[c]

## KEYWORDS

- Key pinch • Lateral pinch • Tip pinch • Power pinch • Ulnar nerve • Tendon transfers • Pinchplasty

## KEY POINTS

- In ulnar nerve paralysis, power pinch is significantly affected and can lead to difficulty with performing daily tasks.
- When nonoperative treatment fails, tendon transfers may be used.
- The primary muscle for power pinch is the adductor pollicis (AP), and secondary muscles are the first dorsal interosseous (DI) and the deep head of the flexor pollicis brevis (FBP).
- Preferred tendon transfers are extensor carpi radialis brevis (ECRB) to AP with z-lengthening for AP restoration, abductor pollicis longus (APL) to first DI tendon transfer using tendon graft for first DI restoration and splin flexor pollicis longus (FPL) to extensor pollicis longus (EPL) transfer thumb stabilization.
- Combinations of transfers should be evaluated on an individual basis.

## INTRODUCTION

### Anatomy

The adductor pollicis (AP) has the largest mass and cross-sectional diameter of any hand intrinsic muscle.[1] It is also able to produce the most force and work capacity of all the intrinsics.[2] It is composed of transverse and oblique heads, which are innervated by the deep branch of the ulnar nerve. The transverse head originates from the third metacarpal and inserts on the ulnar aspect of the thumb proximal phalanx and continues into the lateral bands. The oblique head shares its insertion with the transverse head by a conjoint tendon that attaches to the ulnar sesamoid bone of the thumb but originates from multiple locations. This includes the palmar aspects of the second and third metacarpals, the capitate, the intercarpal ligaments, and the flexor carpi radialis sheath. Together, the transverse and oblique heads contribute to thumb carpometacarpal (CMC)

flexion and adduction, metacarpal phalangeal (MP) flexion, interphalangeal (IP) extension, and thumb supination. The deep head of the flexor pollicis brevis (FPB), also innervated by the deep branch of the ulnar nerve, runs almost parallel to the AP and mimics its function. Between the 2 heads of the AP, the deep motor branch of the ulnar nerve runs along with the radial artery, which course from dorsal to palmar to become the deep arch.[3]

The first dorsal interosseous (DI) muscle is the second largest intrinsic muscle of the hand in terms of mass and cross-sectional area.[1] It is a bipennate muscle, nearly always innervated by the ulnar nerve that originates from the radial side of the second metacarpal and the proximal ulnar aspect of the first metacarpal. The insertion is on the radial aspect of the base of the index finger proximal phalanx and into the radial lateral band.[3] Its primary action is to abduct the index finger, but it also assists the lumbrical in MP joint flexion and

[a] University of Iowa Hospitals and Clinics, 200 Hawkins Drive, 01008 JPP, Iowa City, IA 52242, USA; [b] OrthoCarolina, 1915 Randolph Road, Charlotte, NC 28207, USA; [c] The Hand and Upper Extremity Center of Georgia, PC, Northside/Alpharetta Medical Campus, Suite 350, 3400A Old Milton Parkway, Alpharetta, GA 30005, USA
* Corresponding author.
E-mail address: scook72@gmail.com

Hand Clin 32 (2016) 369–376
http://dx.doi.org/10.1016/j.hcl.2016.03.007
0749-0712/15/$ – see front matter © 2016 Elsevier Inc. All rights reserved.

IP joint extension. Similar to the AP, the low fiber length/muscle length (FL/ML) ratio of DI makes it suitable to provide a large amount of force to allow for power pinch.[1] Together, the AP and DI contribute 75% of the adduction force of the thumb.

The FPB is a weak contributor to power pinch, as it has only one-third the work capacity, force, and mass of the AP.[1,2] The superficial (lateral) head, innervated by the recurrent motor branch of the median nerve, originates from the trapezium and the distal edge of the transverse carpal ligament and inserts on the radial aspect of the base of the thumb proximal phalanx and radial sesamoid. The deep (medial) head, innervated by the ulnar nerve, inserts on the ulnar aspect of the thumb proximal phalanx base along with the AP. The FBP assists in flexion at the MP joint of the thumb along with CMC flexion and IP extension.[3] Innervation can be variable with both heads being supplied by either the median or ulnar nerve or have dual innervation.[4]

### Etiology of Ulnar Nerve Neuropathy

Etiology of ulnar neuropathy can be multifactorial and a broad differential must be considered by the surgeon. Ulnar neuropathy may be due to mechanical cause or systemic pathology. Metabolic derangements, such as diabetes and hypothyroidism, are common causes of generalized neuropathy and should be evaluated. In addition, hereditary neuropathies, such as Charcot-Marie-Tooth, commonly affect the ulnar nerve.[5] Mechanical causes of ulnar neuropathy are often compressive in nature and vary based on anatomic location. Ulnar nerve palsy is generally classified as high or low. Low ulnar nerve palsy is due to an injury at the wrist, whereas high ulnar nerve palsy injury is at the level of the elbow or above, affecting flexor carpi ulnaris (FCU) and flexor digitorum profundus (FDP) to the ring and small finger. Some mechanical etiologies of ulnar nerve palsies include the following:

1. At or near the elbow
   a. Compressive neuropathy (eg, cubital tunnel syndrome)
   b. Penetrating or blunt trauma
   c. Deformities (ie, cubital valgus)
   d. Rheumatoid arthritis
   e. Hemophilia leading to hematomas
   f. Subdermal contraceptive implants
   g. Compression during general anesthesia
   h. Previous elbow surgery (both open and arthroscopic)
2. Near the wrist or distal
   a. Compressive neuropathy

   b. Ganglion cysts
   c. Tumors
   d. Penetrating or blunt trauma
   e. Ulnar artery aneurysm

Clinicians should also consider local clinical conditions at the thumb and index finger as causes for alterations in a patient's pinch that is not due to ulnar nerve dysfunction. This includes congenital anomalies, previous trauma, inflammatory or osteoarthritis, and intrinsic/extrinsic muscle/tendon abnormalities. Last, more proximal nerve compression, such as lower trunk brachial plexopathy, cervical radiculopathy, or a Pancoast tumor, should be considered in the differential diagnosis.

### Pathoanatomy

In patients with ulnar nerve paralysis, the main complaint is loss of effective power pinch and coordination between the thumb and index finger.[6] This can be exaggerated or minimized based on the location of the lesion and anatomic variations of innervation of the hand musculature (ie, Martin-Gruber or Riche-Cannieu cross-innervation patterns). In addition, dysfunction of the ulnar nerve can also lead to dyskinetic finger flexion and deformity such as claw hand, loss of active digital abduction/adduction including persistent little finger abduction, thumb interphalangeal joint hyperflexion, metacarpophalangeal joint hyperextension and severe interossei muscle wasting (Fig. 1). In complete high or low ulnar nerve palsy the only remaining adductors of the thumb are the extensor pollicis longus (EPL), extensor pollicis brevis (EPB), and the flexor pollicis longus (FPL), all which create a weak adduction force. Thus, lesions of both the ulnar and median nerve lead to

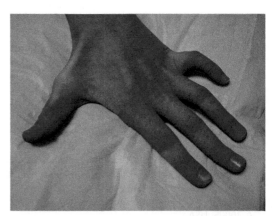

Fig. 1. A clinical photograph of a patient with an ulnar nerve palsy. Atrophy of the first DI and intrinsics is noted with abduction of the small finger and clawing.

a severely compromised pinch.[7] Power pinch can be reduced by more than 80% in patients with an ulnar nerve palsy.[8] There is great variation in force needed to achieve activities of daily living using power pinch. Inserting a plug into an outlet can take as much as 31.4 Newtons (N), whereas as little as 1.4 N is needed to push a button on a remote control.[6] Therefore, tasks such as holding utensils to eat, manipulating buttons while getting dressed, tearing open packages, plugging plugs into outlets, and writing can become difficult to accomplish for patients with an ulnar nerve palsy.

There are numerous eponyms to describe the clinical signs of ulnar nerve palsy. Signs that are specific to pinch include Jeanne sign (hyperextension of the thumb MP joint with pinch) and Froment sign (pronounced flexion of the IP joint of the thumb with pinch).[8] There is significant individual variability in terms of tolerance of this functional deficit with some patients quite functional and satisfied with their pinch capabilities, despite significant weakness and others significantly affected.

Interestingly, with today's technology, a positive Froment sign may be advantageous from a positional standpoint, as IP joint flexion is frequently used for cellular devices.[9] From a mechanical standpoint, however, IP joint hyperflexion results in loss of pinch power. A heavy laborer, therefore, may tremendously benefit from an IP fusion or FPL splin transfer, whereas other patients with lower strength requirements and specific vocational positional needs can find this loss of IP flexion frustrating. Therefore, surgical augmentation of power pinch must be individualized. If uncertainty exists, a temporary IP pinning can be helpful in some cases as a trial for the patient.

## Treatment

When the potential for nerve recovery and muscle strength have been maximized, and weakness in pinch remains a functional limitation, surgical intervention should be considered. Surgery should focus primarily on restoring adduction of the thumb. Restoring abduction of the index finger and/or stabilizing the thumb and index finger needs to be evaluated on a case-by-case basis. Often we have found tendon transfers for abduction of the index finger are unnecessary, as the long, ring, and small fingers can provide an anatomic post for the index finger for power pinch.

Basic principles of tendon transfer should always be followed, which include consideration of the donor tendon strength and excursion, vector of pull, surrounding soft tissue conditions, preoperative joint range of motion, and in-phase function of the donor and recipient actions.[10] Once these factors have been considered, then surgical intervention can be planned. When planning for restoration of pinch, the surgeon must consider the possibility of staged procedures to correct other abnormalities seen in ulnar neuropathy, such as dyskinetic grasp. We typically will choose a palmar muscle for one transfer and a dorsal muscle for the other when staging pinch and grasp reconstruction. Contraindications to surgery include stiffness or contractures, poor soft tissues, lack of patient compliance with postoperative compliance and rehabilitation, and a progressive neurologic condition.[11]

## SURGICAL TECHNIQUES
### Restoration of Thumb Adduction

Restoration of thumb adduction is the most important undertaking for recreating power pinch. To restore adduction of the thumb, augmentation of the transverse head of the AP should be the primary focus. As previously noted, the AP is the largest and strongest intrinsic muscle in the hand and therefore needs a strong motor donor to restore pinch strength. Many tendon transfers to restore pinch have been described in the literature (**Box 1**). The ideal vector for restoring pinch should be in line with the fibers of the transverse head of the AP. Tendon transfers that instead parallel the fibers of the deep head of the FPB and oblique head of the AP and/or EPL provide very minimal improvement and are not recommended. In addition, muscles with inadequate strength are not suitable for transfer (eg, extensor indicis proprius [EIP] and extensor digiti minimi [EDM]). Considering the necessary strength and excursion, it is our preference to use the extensor carpi radialis brevis (ECRB) for restoration of pinch. This transfer has been most often

---

**Box 1**
**Restoration of thumb adduction**

- Flexor digitorum superficialis (FDS) ring finger or middle finger to adductor[15]
- Extensor carpi radialis brevis (ECRB) with tendon graft through third intermetacarpal space to adductor[12]
- Brachioradialis (BR) to adductor[16]
- Extensor indicis proprius (EIP) to adductor[16]
- Split extensor digiti minimi (EDM) to adductor[17]
- Extensor digitorum communis (EDC) to index finger to adductor[18]

described using a tendon graft to provide the necessary length for the tendon transfer, but the authors' preference is to perform a long Z-plasty of ECRB without the use of a tendon graft (**Fig. 2**B). Hastings and Davidson[7] and Smith[12] showed that the ECRB adductorplasty (using tendon graft) increased the preoperative pinch strength twofold.

In cases of concomitant radial nerve palsy or when a planned use of the ECRB for restoration of grasp is planned, we prefer to use the flexor digitorum superficialis (FDS) of the ring or long finger as a donor tendon. Either the middle finger or ring finger FDS may be used in low ulnar nerve palsy,[13,14] but in high ulnar nerve palsy, only the middle finger FDS should be used, as the FDS is the sole remaining digital flexor of the ring finger. FDS transfers have been shown to improve pinch strength 30% to 70%. Because of the more favorable soft tissue bed, in contrast to the ECRB transfer, tenolysis is rarely required. This transfer also carries the benefit of not requiring a graft or

lengthening. A full list of described donor tendons for restoration of pinch is in **Box 1**.

## SURGICAL TECHNIQUE
### Extensor Carpi Radialis Brevis to Adductor Pollicis Muscle Tendon Transfer

- A transverse incision is made over the third metacarpal base.
- Release the ECRB off the radial aspect of the third metacarpal base.
- Make a second incision proximal to dorsal wrist extensor retinaculum.
- Deliver the ECRB through this proximal incision (**Fig. 2**A).
- Make a third incision at the ulnar base of the thumb MP joint.
- A free tendon autograft (palmaris longus [PL] or half of flexor carpi radialis [FCR]) is passed from the thumb incision between the AP and interossei volar to the second metacarpal bone and dorsally out between the second

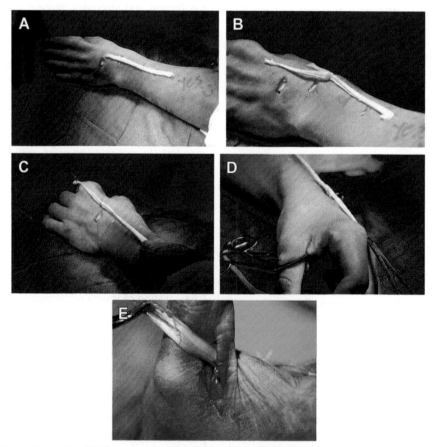

**Fig. 2.** ECRB to AP transfer. (*A*) Harvesting the ECRB through multiple transverse incisions. (*B*) Z-lengthening of the ECRB. (*C*) Distal suture applied into the z-lengthened tendon (*D*) using a curved tendon passer to pass the ECRB into the AP insertion. (*E*) Passing the ECRB into the AP insertion along the ulnar border of the thumb MP joint.

and third or third and fourth metacarpal bones using a curved tendon passer (**Fig. 2D**).

- Alternatively, a long z-lengthening of the ECRB can be performed and routed in the same manner (**Fig. 2B**) as this is the authors' preferred method.
- Suture the free graft to the AP tendon at its insertion.
- The wrist is held in neutral with the thumb adducted against the index finger.
- If a free graft is used, a Pulvertaft weave is performed, suturing the proximal end of the tendon to the ECRB.
- Make sure ECRB is at its mid-excursion length (half way between resting length and maximal excursion) before suturing.
- The same tensioning principles are followed for distal attachment of a z-lengthened ECRB into the AP.
- Passively flex and extend the wrist to test thumb abduction/adduction tension.
- Firm adduction of the thumb against the index finger should be present with passive wrist flexion.
- Full abduction of the thumb should be present with passive wrist extension.
- With the thumb in neutral, the thumb should lay just volar to the index ray.
- Once proper tension has been achieved, the tendon graft is Pulvertaft woven 3 times through the ECRB tendon.
- If the patient has weak opposition, slightly less tension should be applied.
- Thumb spica splint for 4 weeks with the thumb in neutral position and the wrist in 30 to 40° of extension.
- At 4 weeks, begin gentle active and active assisted range of motion exercises and transition to a forearm-based thumb spica splint.
- At 8 to 10 weeks, begin resistive pinch and grip.
- At 3 to 4 months, can resume all but high-demand activities, and at 6 months, return to activity as tolerated.

- Occasionally a tenolysis is required at the pulley point around the metacarpal.

### Flexor Digitorum Superficialis III or IV to Adductor Pollicis Muscle Tendon Transfer

- Make an oblique skin incision centered over the A1 pulley.
- Release the A1 pulley and apply maximal traction to the FDS.
- Transect tendon just proximal to the decussation.
- Use the vertical septum of the superficial palmar fascia attached to the second metacarpal as a pulley when the middle finger FDS is used.
- Make an incision of the ulnar side of the thumb MP joint.
- Tunnel the FDS subcutaneously toward the AP tendon insertion.
- Suture the tendon to the AP tendon insertion with the tension set with the wrist at 30° of extension with the thumb adducted against the index finger.
- Firm adduction should be present with passive wrist extension and full abduction with maximal passive wrist flexion (**Fig. 3**).
- Thumb spica splint for 4 weeks.
- At 4 weeks, begin gentle active and active assisted range of motion exercises and transition to a forearm-based thumb spica splint.
- At 8 to 10 weeks, begin resistive pinch and grip.
- At 3 to 4 months, can resume all but high-demand activities, and at 6 months, return to activity as tolerated.

### Restoration of Index Finger Abduction

In addition to restoring the adduction moment of the AP, it is important to evaluate if the patient would benefit from restoration of index finger abduction in augmenting pinch. The goal of this potential tendon transfer is to make the index finger serve as a post and avoid ulnar deviation

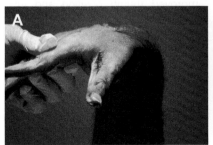
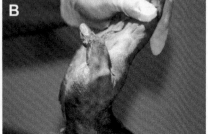

**Fig. 3.** Tensioning the FDS transfer to AP. (*A*) Passive wrist flexion resulting on full thumb abduction. (*B*) Passive wrist flexion resulting in full thumb abduction.

of the digit under load. Several tendon transfers have been described in the literature, as can be seen in **Box 2**. The authors' preferred treatment is abductor pollicis longus (APL) slip to the first DI via tendon autograft. In our experience, this transfer is not commonly needed, as most patients compensate well bracing the index finger against the adjacent fingers with pinch. The individual's pattern of pinch should be observed preoperatively to assess the need for this transfer. Using slips of extensor carpi radialis longus (ECRL) to AP and first DI transfer, Fischer and colleagues[19] showed the mean force of index finger abduction was 58% of the unaffected side. Mean key pinch was 73% of the unaffected side. Yet, it is the authors' experience that transfers using overly powerful donor tendons (ECRL) can lead to unwanted fixed abduction of the index finger, because the EIP is the only remaining adduction force of the digit given the paralysis of the first volar interosseous.

## SURGICAL TECHNIQUE
### Abductor Pollicis Longus to First Dorsal Interosseous Muscle Tendon Transfer

- Make an incision over the insertion of the APL on the first metacarpal base.
- Detach one slip of the APL from its insertion.
- Transfer the slip proximally out of the first compartment pulley and pass it subcutaneously toward the first DI tendon.
- Lengthen the APL slip with free tendon graft (preferably PL).
- Suture the tendon graft to the DI tendon insertion palmer to the axis of rotation.
- Using a Pulvertaft weave, connect the graft to the APL slip.[21]
- Tension the graft with the index finger abducted maximally and the APL at half maximal excursion.
- An intrinsic-plus radial-gutter forearm-based splint is applied for 4 weeks.
- Active range of motion is begun at 4 weeks.

- Passive range of motion is begun at 8 weeks, as well as light strengthening.
- Power grip and pinch is allowed at 3 months.

### Thumb Metacarpal Phalangeal and Interphalangeal Joint Stabilization

The final step of restoring a competent pinch is to stabilize the IP and MP joints of the thumb. The MP and IP joints collapse into predictable patterns of deformity in the presence of ulnar nerve palsy. The loss of multiple MP flexors (AP and FPB) leads to a force imbalance favoring MP hyperextension, and once the stout volar plate attenuates over time, a resting MP hyperextension deformity (known as a Jeanne sign) may develop. Simultaneously, the IP joint sees a loss of extension power from the weakness of intrinsic contribution to IP extension and a reciprocal flexion deformity develops as the FPL is recruited to augment adduction strength resulting in the Froment sign. The IP flexion and MP hyperextension deformities place the thumb at a significant mechanical disadvantage and result in a further weakening of pinch due to the inability to normally distribute forces across these joints. Surgical stabilization of these joints can markedly improve force distribution and thus pinch strength. These changes in joint position should be discussed preoperatively, though, as some patients now enjoy the IP flexion in particular that is required for texting and operation of small electronic devices. Therefore, careful patient selection is mandated for thumb stabilization.

If persistent MP hyperextension and IP hyperflexion remain following tendon transfer for adduction, several options are available, as seen in **Box 3**. The authors' preferred method is a FPL split to EPL transfer or IP versus MP joint arthrodesis depending on the patient's demands. Van Heest and colleagues[22] showed that 12 split FPL transfers in 10 patients completely eliminated the Froment sign and limited IP joint flexion to between 15° to 30°. All patients had full IP joint extension and all patients were satisfied with improved thumb position and function. An IP fusion alone results in an average of 2 kg improvement in pinch strength, yet the loss of dexterity must be considered. An MP fusion

---

**Box 2**
**Restoration of index finger abduction**

- Accessory abductor pollicis longus (APL) to first dorsal interosseous (DI)[19]
- Extensor carpi radialis longus (ECRL) to first DI via index EDC graft
- EIP to first dorsal interosseous[17]
- Palmaris longus (PL) with extension to first dorsal interosseous[20]

---

**Box 3**
**Thumb stabilization**

- Partial flexor pollicis longus (FPL) to extensor pollicis longus (EPL) transfer[23]
- Metacarpal phalangeal (MP) and/or interphalangeal (IP) joint arthrodesis

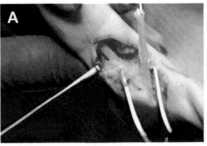
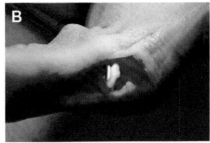

**Fig. 4.** The split FPL to EPL transfer. (*A*) The radial half of the FPL is split longitudinal from its distal insertion and retracted proximal to the oblique pulley. (*B*) It is then passed deep to the neurovascular bundle and wrapped around the EPL and back to itself.

reliably corrects the Jeanne sign; however, this does not always simultaneously correct the Froment sign and sometimes this must be addressed in a subsequent procedure. Like the IP fusion, an MP fusion results in an average gain of 2 kg of pinch strength. The optimal position for MP fusion is 15° of flexion, 5° of abduction, and 15° of pronation. When performing an MP fusion, release of the flexor pulleys proximally can allow slight bowstringing of the tendons to further enhance pinch power.

## SURGICAL TECHNIQUE
### *Split Flexor Pollicis Longus to Extensor Pollicis Longus Transfer*

- Make a mid-lateral incision along the radial border of the thumb to provide access to FPL.
- Split the FPL at the natural longitudinal seam.
- Release the radial half of the FPL tendon at its insertion.
- Deliver proximal to the oblique pulley (**Fig. 4**A).
- Make a dorsal midline incision over the IP joint to expose the EPL.
- Pass the radial slip of the FPL around the radial aspect of the thumb between the first annular pulley and the oblique pulley deep to the neurovascular bundle.
- Bring the FPL under the EPL and wrap it over the top of the EPL and back onto itself (**Fig. 4**B).
- Fix the IP joint in slight flexion using a Kirschner wire.
- Tension the FPL so there is equal tension on both the ulnar and radial slips and for pulp-to-pulp contact between the thumb and index finger with tip pinch.
- Secure with nonabsorbable suture.
- Immobilize the thumb for 4 weeks.
- Remove Kirschner wire at 5 to 6 weeks.
- Project IP joint for a total of 8 weeks.

## SUMMARY

The primary muscle for power pinch is the AP and secondary muscles are the first DI and the deep head of the FBP. In ulnar nerve paralysis, power pinch is significantly affected and can lead to difficult with performing activities of daily living and other tasks. When nonoperative treatment fails, tendon transfers may be used. The authors' preferred tendon transfers are ECRB to AP with z-lengthening for AP restoration, APL to first DI tendon transfer using tendon graft for first DI restoration, and splin FPL to EPL transfer thumb stabilization. Combinations of transfers should be evaluated on an individual basis.

## REFERENCES

1. Jacobson MD, Raab R, Fazeli BM, et al. Architectural design of the human intrinsic hand muscles. J Hand Surg Am 1992;17(5):804–9.
2. Fahrer M. The thenar eminence: an introduction. Hand 1981;1:255–8.
3. Thompson JC. Netter's concise orthopaedic anatomy. Philadelphia: Elsevier Health Sciences; 2009.
4. Day M, Napier J. The two heads of flexor pollicis brevis. J Anat 1961;95(Pt 1):123.
5. Auer-Grumbach M, Wagner K, Strasser-Fuchs S, et al. Clinical predominance of proximal upper limb weakness in CMT1A syndrome. Muscle Nerve 2000;23(8):1243–9.
6. Smaby N, Johanson ME, Baker B, et al. Identification of key pinch forces required to complete functional tasks. J Rehabil Res Dev 2004;41(2):215.
7. Hastings H 2nd, Davidson S. Tendon transfers for ulnar nerve palsy. Evaluation of results and practical treatment considerations. Hand Clin 1988;4(2):167–78.
8. Mannerfelt L. Studies on the hand in ulnar nerve paralysis: a clinical-experimental investigation in normal and anomalous innervation. Acta Orthop Scand 1966;37(Suppl 87):3–176.
9. Jonsson P, Johnson PW, Hagberg M, et al. Thumb joint movement and muscular activity during

mobile phone texting: a methodological study. J Electromyogr Kinesiol 2011;21(2):363–70.

10. Seiler JG III, Desai MJ, Payne HS. Tendon transfers for radial, median, and ulnar nerve palsy. J Am Acad Orthop Surg 2013;21(11):675–84.

11. Tse R, Hentz VR, Yao J. Late reconstruction for ulnar nerve palsy. Hand Clin 2007;23(3):373–92, vii.

12. Smith RJ. Extensor carpi radialis brevis tendon transfer for thumb adduction—a study of power pinch. J Hand Surg Am 1983;8(1):4–15.

13. North ER, Littler JW. Transferring the flexor superficialis tendon: technical considerations in the prevention of proximal interphalangeal joint disability. J Hand Surg Am 1980;5(5):498–501.

14. Lee SK, Wisser JR. Restoration of pinch in intrinsic muscles of the hand. Hand Clin 2012;28(1):45–51.

15. Goldner J. Tendon transfers for irreparable peripheral nerve injuries of the upper extremity. Orthop Clin North Am 1974;5(2):343.

16. Edgerton MT, Brand PW. Restoration of the abduction and the adduction to the unstable thumb in median and ulnar nerve paralysis. Plast Reconstr Surg 1965;36(2):150–64.

17. Robinson D, Aghasi MK, Halperin N. Restoration of pinch in ulnar nerve palsy by transfer of split extensor digiti minimi and extensor indicis. J Hand Surg Br 1992;17(6):622–4.

18. Boyes JH. Bunnell's surgery of the hand. Acad Med 1964;39(9):871.

19. Fischer T, Nagy L, Buechler U. Restoration of pinch grip in ulnar nerve paralysis: extensor carpi radialis longus to adductor pollicis and abductor pollicis longus to first dorsal interosseus tendon transfers. J Hand Surg Br 2003;28(1):28–32.

20. Hirayama T, Atsuta Y, Takemitsu Y. Palmaris longus transfer for replacement of the first dorsal interosseous. J Hand Surg Br 1986;11(1):84–6.

21. Neviaser RJ, Wilson JN, Gardner MM. Abductor pollicis longus transfer for replacement of first dorsal interosseous. J Hand Surg 1980;5(1):53–7.

22. Van Heest A, Hanson D, Lee J, et al. Split flexor pollicus longus tendon transfer for stabilization of the thumb interphalangeal joint: a cadaveric and clinical study. J Hand Surg 1999;24(6):1303–10.

23. Mohammed KD, Rothwell AG, Sinclair SW, et al. Upper-limb surgery for tetraplegia. J Bone Joint Surg Br 1992;74(6):873–9.

# Tendon Transfers for Combined Peripheral Nerve Injuries

Christopher A. Makarewich, MD,
Douglas T. Hutchinson, MD*

## KEYWORDS

- Tendon transfer • Combined • Nerve • Injury • Palsy • Median • Ulnar • Radial

## KEY POINTS

- Tendon transfers for combined nerve injuries have significant limitations due to available muscle tendon units, scarring, and the significant rehabilitation required.
- Surgical reconstruction must be individualized with a focus on restoring functional goals.
- The suggestions in this article should only be considered as a rough guide, because some may be reasonable and others not in a given patient.

## INTRODUCTION

Combined peripheral nerve injuries present a unique set of challenges to the hand surgeon when considering tendon transfers. Typically they result from severe trauma to the upper extremity and can be associated with significant injuries to soft tissue, bone, and vascular structures.[1] Muscle and tendon injuries requiring repair may both worsen motor deficits and limit the number of viable tendons available for transfer. Significant scar formation can complicate reconstruction due to adhesion formation, increasing the difficulty of establishing a reasonable path for tendon rerouting. In addition, the accompanying sensory deficits are often more severe than single nerve injuries with profound loss of both protective and fine sensation, making function not simply a matter of repositioning and muscle transfer.[1,2]

These sensory deficits have been suggested as the most critical factor in determining overall hand function.[1,3,4] Protective sensation of pain and temperature is lost as well as the ability for the hand and digits to identify their place in 3-dimensional space (proprioception). There is a close association between motor function and sensation, and abnormal patterns of motor activity can worsen these sensory deficits.[3] It has been suggested that tendon transfers should be completed before attempts to improve sensation,[1] although they can be combined in one sitting for the convenience of the patient if the tendon transfer rehabilitation is not compromised. The restoration of sensation can be attempted through direct nerve repair, nerve grafting, nerve transfer, and skin and tissue transplants to key areas of sensation, including the radial and ulnar borders of the thumb, radial border of the index, and ulnar border of the hand.[1,5–7] Unfortunately, in many cases of combined peripheral nerve injuries, if return of sensation is not anticipated, tendon transfers are not indicated.[1,2]

The general principles of tendon transfers have been well described earlier in this issue as well as elsewhere[2,8–10]; however, there are specific considerations related to combined nerve palsies. Donor muscle tendon units (MTUs) (**Table 1**) must be of normal or near normal strength (at least 4/5),

Disclosure Statement: No disclosures.
Department of Orthopaedics, University of Utah, 590 Wakara Way, Room A0100, Salt Lake City, UT 84108, USA
* Corresponding author.
*E-mail address:* Douglas.Hutchinson@hsc.utah.edu

Hand Clin 32 (2016) 377–387
http://dx.doi.org/10.1016/j.hcl.2016.03.008

**Table 1**
**Muscle tendon unit abbreviations**

| Abbreviation | Muscle Name |
|---|---|
| ADM | Abductor digiti minimi |
| APB | Abductor pollicis brevis |
| BR | Brachioradialis |
| ECRB | Extensor carpi radialis brevis |
| ECRL | Extensor carpi radialis longus |
| ECU | Extensor carpi ulnaris |
| EDC | Extensor digitorum communis |
| EDM | Extensor digiti minimi |
| EIP | Extensor indicis proprius |
| EPL | Extensor pollicis longus |
| FCR | Flexor carpi radialis |
| FCU | Flexor carpi ulnaris |
| FDP | Flexor digitorum profundus |
| FDS | Flexor digitorum superficialis |
| FPB | Flexor pollicis brevis |
| FPL | Flexor pollicis longus |
| PL | Palmaris longus |
| PT | Pronator teres |

have similar excursion, and preferably act in phase with the recipient tendon. Tendon transfers rely on the redundant action of multiple tendons, making some tendons expendable for donors without loss of function. In the case of combined nerve injuries, there are typically fewer options for transfer because of fewer tendons of shared function that are expendable as well as associated injuries to tendon or muscle bellies. Careful preoperative planning must be performed to make the most of remaining MTUs (**Table 2**). Before considering transfer, tissue equilibrium should be complete with wounds and fractures healed, and full passive range of motion should be achieved. In addition to tendon transfers, joint arthrodesis should be considered in certain cases, more so with combined nerve injuries than single nerve injuries, both to improve function and to provide additional tendons for transfer.

Particularly in combined nerve injuries, the goal of tendon transfer is to restore function rather than replace specific muscle groups.[1,9] It is important for the surgeon to establish the goals of care with the patient, with the understanding of both parties that it will not be possible to re-create a

**Table 2**
**Anatomic deficits, reconstructive goals, and available muscle tendon units for transfer in combined peripheral nerve injuries**

| Combined Nerve Injury | Anatomic Deficits | Reconstructive Goals | Available MTUs for Transfer |
|---|---|---|---|
| Low median-ulnar | All hand intrinsics | • Key pinch<br>• Thumb opposition<br>• Treatment of clawing<br>• Coordinated MP and IP joint flexion | • Radial innervated muscle groups (BR and all extensors)<br>• PT, FCR, FPL, FDS, FCU, PL |
| High median-ulnar | • All hand intrinsics<br>• External finger flexors<br>• Finger flexors | • Key pinch<br>• Thumb opposition<br>• Finger flexion for simple grip<br>• Treatment of clawing<br>• Coordinated MP and IP joint flexion | Radial innervated muscle groups (BR and all extensors) |
| High ulnar-radial | • Hypothenar muscles<br>• Ulnar intrinsics<br>• Finger and wrist extensors<br>• Ulnar half of FDP | • Wrist extension<br>• Finger and thumb extension<br>• Thumb adduction<br>• Ring and small finger flexion | • PT, FCR, PL, FDS<br>• Radial half FDP |
| High median-radial | • All wrist MTUs *except* FCU<br>• All extrinsic finger flexors and extensors<br>• Thenar muscles *except* adductor pollicis and deep portion FPB | • Thumb opposition<br>• Mass action grip<br>• Thumb and finger extension | • FCU after wrist arthrodesis<br>• Ulnar half FDP<br>• Hypothenar muscles |

normal hand. The uninjured hand will take up the task of fine-motor skills, while the goal for the injured hand is to create the most useful helper hand possible.[1] To accomplish this, the need for an individualized approach is essential, with tendon transfers planned to fulfill the patient's specific functional needs. In addition, critical considerations include the postoperative course and anticipated rehabilitation protocols. The patient has to be available for likely multiple times-per-week hand therapy or the outcomes may be poor enough to contraindicate the surgery in the first place. Transfers should only be performed simultaneously if they can be rehabilitated together, a challenge that sometimes necessitates a staged approach with multiple procedures.

## LOW MEDIAN-ULNAR NERVE PALSY

Anatomic deficits
- Loss of all hand intrinsics

Reconstructive goals
- Key pinch, thumb opposition, treatment of clawing, coordinated metacarpophalangeal joint (MPJ), and interphalangeal joint (IPJ) flexion

Available MTUs
- Radial innervated muscle groups (brachioradialis [BR] and all extensors)
- Pronator teres (PT), flexor carpi radialis (FCR), flexor pollicis longus (FPL), flexor digitorum superficialis (FDS), flexor digitorum profundus (FDP), flexor carpi ulnaris (FCU), palmaris longus (PL)

The low median-ulnar palsy is the most common combined peripheral nerve injury, typically due to a volar laceration of the wrist.[2] As a result of this mechanism, donor tendon selection may be limited due to concomitant laceration of the extrinsic flexor tendons. In addition to entire loss of palmar sensation, loss of both median and ulnar innervated muscle groups in the hand leads to asynchronous finger flexion and clawing of the digits as well as loss of key pinch and opposition.[1,2,9] Restoration of each of these functions is approached as follows.

### Key Pinch

Key pinch results from the combined action of adductor pollicis and first dorsal interosseous muscles, both of which are lost in the low median-ulnar palsy. Techniques to reproduce both of these functions simultaneously have

been described[11]; however, typically it is only necessary to restore adductor pollicis function because the index finger can be braced against the remaining digits. The most successful transfers involve a direct line of pull transversely across the palm, inserting on the adductor pollicis tendon.[4,12,13] Described donor tendons include extensor carpi radialis brevis (ECRB), extensor carpi radialis longus (ECRL), BR, and FDS.

ECRB transfer with tendon graft is the preferred method in combined median-ulnar nerve palsies **(Fig. 1)**.[1,13,14] In this technique, the ECRB tendon is harvested at its insertion and lengthened with a tendon graft or long z-plasty, which can then be passed through the second or third intermetacarpal space and inserted on the adductor pollicis

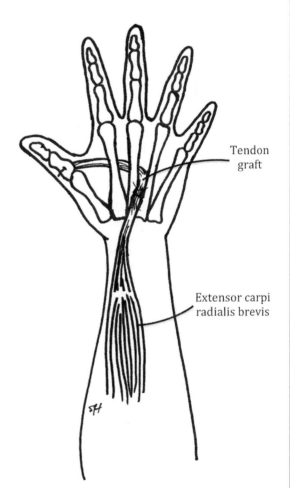

Tendon graft

Extensor carpi radialis brevis

**Fig. 1.** Reconstruction of thumb adduction using ECRB. ECRB is extended with tendon graft and passed dorsal to palmar between metacarpals 3 and 4. This interval avoids the potentially scarred adductor pollicis, which originates in part of the third metacarpal. The tendon is then attached to the adductor pollicis insertion.

tendon. The second or third metacarpal then acts as a pulley to re-create the adductor pollicis' anatomic direction of pull. Placing the graft through the space between the third and fourth metacarpals avoids the potentially scarred adductor pollicis, which originates in part of the third metacarpal. Proper tensioning of this transfer is difficult because if placed too tight it can compromise the first web space and decrease function. Because of this, some choose to avoid this transfer and use the MTU for other purposes.

Consideration for IPJ stabilization also needs to be made in this injury pattern to prevent the inefficient Froment pinch. In the unbalanced thumb with an intact extrinsic flexor (FPL) and loss of intrinsic thumb muscle balance, thumb flexion can lead to intercalated collapse and IPJ hyperflexion (Froment sign) with loss of the stronger pulp pinch. To correct this, the FPL can be split with the radial half transferred dorsally and woven into the EPL at the level of the proximal phalanx.[15] Should severe MPJ hyperextension (Jeanne sign) be present, arthrodesis of the joint may be necessary to restore strong pinch.[16]

### Thumb Opposition

Thumb opposition is a critical hand motion that requires special consideration. It is affected by all combined injuries that involve the median nerve, and its restoration is a major reconstructive goal to produce a functional hand. Opposition is a complex motion involving abduction, pronation, and flexion at the carpometacarpal joint, abduction and flexion at the MPJ, and either flexion or extension at the IPJ; this brings the pulp of the thumb in contact with the terminal pad of the index finger to allow for precise grasping of objects. There are several donor tendons available to restore this function, the selection of which can be tailored based on the muscles affected. Options include extensor indicis proprius (EIP),[17] ring-finger FDS through a distal based slip of FCU,[18] PL extended with a strip of palmar fascia,[19,20] extensor digiti minimi (EDM),[21] and extensor carpi ulnaris (ECU) sutured to a distal slip of extensor pollicis brevis.[22] Regardless of choice of donor tendon, the techniques share similar principles. To be effective, transfers should pull in line with the pisiform (often requiring the construction of a pulley) and insert onto the dorsal and radial aspect of the proximal phalanx of the thumb.[18,23] Although several specific insertion points have been described, the abductor pollicis brevis (APB) is generally accepted as the ideal target, permitting full abduction and pronation as confirmed in a 1984 biomechanical study.[24] Some have suggested however

that in combined median and ulnar palsies in which all intrinsic muscle balance is lost that insertion into the APB and EPL tendons (Riordan) or into the APB dorsal joint capsule and adductor insertion (Brand) is preferred.[12,17,24] By using a combined insertion that includes EPL, there is increased tension on the long extensor, which in turn limits flexion of the IPJ. In this setting as FPL begins to flex the IPJ; it is checked by the tight EPL, and the remainder of FPL excursion will cause MPJ flexion, thus re-creating the action of FPB.[17]

In the case of the low median-ulnar nerve palsy, the authors' preferred technique is the Burkhalter EIP transfer to APB (**Figs. 2** and **3**).[17] First described in 1973, this transfer begins with transecting the EIP tendon just proximal to the index finger MPJ. The tendon is then mobilized and pulled proximally out from under the extensor retinaculum, brought subcutaneously around the ulnar wrist and obliquely distal to the pisiform across the palm, and sutured to the APB tendon at its insertion as well as to the EPL.

### Clawing and Synchronized Flexion

With the loss of hand intrinsics, the fingers take on a claw conformation with hyperextension at the MPJs and flexion of the proximal interphalangeal joint (PIPJ) and distal interphalangeal joints (DIPJ) (**Fig. 4**). Clawing occurs as the interossei act as the main flexors of the MPJs, and when lost, the unopposed pull of the extrinsic extensors leads to hyperextension. The loss of the interosseous muscles further limits extension at the PIPJ and DIPJs, resulting in unopposed flexion by the FDS and FDP. Several approaches to correct this deformity have been described, including transfers of BR, ECRL, ECRB, EIP, EDM, FDS, FCR, and PL.[2,4,12,25] In the combined low median-ulnar nerve injury, the preferred donor MTU is the ECRL or BR, both of which need to be lengthened using 4-tailed tendon or fascia lata graft. As initially described by Brand,[25] ECRL is released from its insertion, tunneled around the radial border of the forearm, and brought deep to the flexor tendons through the carpal tunnel. Each of the 4 strips of graft are then passed palmar to the deep transverse metacarpal ligament through the lumbrical canals to the radial lateral bands of the long, ring, and small fingers and the ulnar lateral band of the index finger or to the combined interosseous tendon insertions. An alternate path is to pass the tendon grafts from dorsal to palmar at the level of the hand through the interosseous spaces, then volar to the transverse intermetacarpal ligament, through the lumbrical canals, and join them to

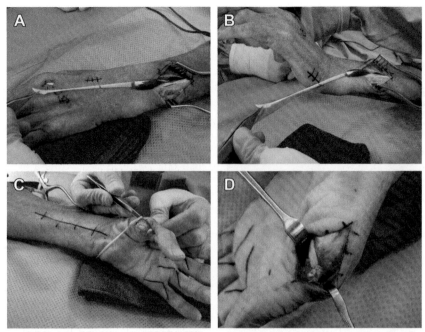

**Fig. 2.** Intraoperative photographs of the EIP opponensplasty. (*A*) The EIP tendon is transected just proximal to the index finger MPJ, (*B*) brought subcutaneously around the ulnar border of the wrist, and (*C*) obliquely distal to the pisiform across the palm, and (*D*) sutured to the APB tendon at its insertion as well as to EPL.

the lateral bands as above.[25] This tendon path has the advantage of avoiding volar scarring. Ideal tensioning has the donor and graft tendons relaxed with wrist at 45° of dorsiflexion, MPJ in 70° of flexion, and IPJ straight.

## HIGH MEDIAN-ULNAR NERVE PALSY

Anatomic deficits
- Loss of all hand intrinsics, extrinsic finger, and wrist flexors

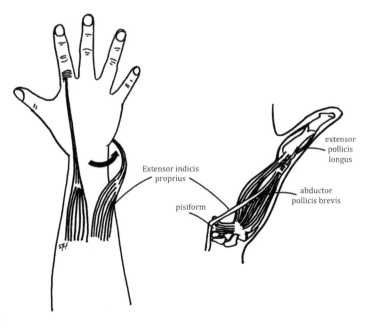

**Fig. 3.** Diagram of the EIP opponensplasty showing rerouting of the EIP tendon and the use of the ulnar side of the hand at the level of the pisiform as a pulley.

extensor
pollicis
longus

Extensor indicis
proprius

abductor
pollicis brevis

pisiform

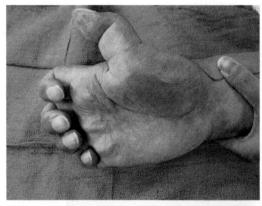

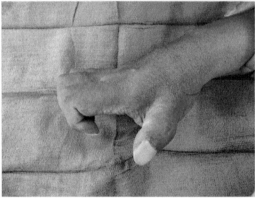

**Fig. 4.** Clawing of the hand with hyperextension at the MPJs and flexion of the PIPJ and DIPJ secondary to palsy of all hand intrinsics.

Reconstructive goals
- Key pinch, thumb opposition, finger flexion for simple grip, treatment of clawing, coordinated MP, and IPJ flexion

Available MTUs
- Radial innervated muscle groups (BR and all extensors)

The more proximal nature of the high median-ulnar nerve palsy creates a significantly greater functional deficit than the low median-ulnar combined injury. The goals of treatment are similar to those of the low median-ulnar palsy described above, including key pinch, thumb opposition, and simple grip, but other concurrent transfers such as those to create finger flexion need to be considered as well.[1]

## Thumb Function

The restoration of thumb opposition and thumb adduction for key pinch can be accomplished as above. The recommended approach is again using ECRB with tendon graft to adductor pollicis

for thumb adduction and the EIP to APB transfer for opposition. However, once again, this transfer might be omitted if another wrist extensor is needed to be used for finger flexion (see later discussion) as one would not want to use both and rely on only ECU to stabilize the wrist. Arthrodesis of the thumb MPJ can help to strengthen both of these actions.[16] To restore thumb IPJ flexion, BR is transferred to the nearby FPL tendon.[26] Other approaches include the split FPL tenodesis[15] as described above, although again this cannot be combined with MPJ arthrodesis because metacarpophalangeal (MP) flexion is required for the tenodesis to be effective.

## Simple Grip and Clawing

Simple grip of the index through small fingers must be addressed differently than in the low median-ulnar palsy where extrinsic flexion is still intact. The typical transfer involves ECRL to the tendons of FDP. ECRL is transected and tunneled subcutaneously around the radial border of the forearm or through the interosseous membrane and sutured to the FDP tendons in the distal forearm proximal to the carpal tunnel. The FDP tendons can be sutured side to side to assist in mass grip. The FPL can be included if BR is unavailable.

Clawing of the digits can occur per the same mechanism as described above. In the high median-ulnar combined injury however, tendon transfer for clawing is not the preferred option due to the limited number of donor tendons. Static and dynamic methods to prevent MPJ hyperextension are the focus. Static methods include the Zancolli volar capsulodesis and tenodesis with tendon graft sutured from the deep transverse intermetacarpal ligament, through the lumbrical canal, and sutured to the extensor mechanism via the lateral bands.[27,28] Dynamic tenodesis options include split tendon graft looped through the wrist extensor retinaculum and taken through a similar path of the static tenodesis along the lumbricals and inserted on the lateral bands of adjacent fingers (**Fig. 5**). Wrist flexion then creates MPJ flexion and PIPJ and DIPJ extension. Arthrodesis has also been described for MP and PIPJs.

With the absence of all wrist flexors, some have considered wrist arthrodesis to allow for transfer of the wrist extensors, including ECRL, ECRB, and ECU. However, this eliminates the possibility of assisted action of dynamic tenodesis through wrist extension, something in general that is required to improve excursion and therefore function.

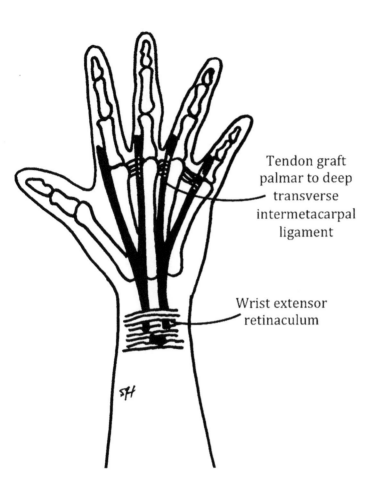

**Fig. 5.** Restoration of synchronized flexion with dynamic tenodesis. Split tendon graft is looped through the wrist extensor retinaculum and taken through the lumbricals and inserted on the radial lateral bands of adjacent fingers.

Tendon graft palmar to deep transverse intermetacarpal ligament

Wrist extensor retinaculum

## HIGH ULNAR-RADIAL NERVE PALSY

Anatomic deficits
- Loss of hypothenar muscles, adductor pollicis, finger and wrist extensors, ulnar half of FDP

Reconstructive goals
- Wrist extension, finger and thumb extension, thumb adduction, ulnar finger flexion

Available MTUs
- PT, PL, FDS, radial half of FDP, FCR

The high ulnar-radial nerve palsy has the benefit of preserved median nerve sensation, making transfers more likely to result in a good functional outcome.[1] It does however generally require a staged approach to reconstruction, as both finger and wrist flexors and extensors need to be recreated and rehabilitated.

### Wrist Extension

Following the approach of Boyes[29] to radial nerve palsy, wrist extension is addressed with PT

transfer to ECRB (**Fig. 6**). PT is released from its insertion along with a periosteal extension and brought subcutaneously around the radial border of the forearm, superficial to the BR and ECRL tendons and joined to ECRB in an end-to-side fashion. Transfer of PT to ECRL has also been described; however, this can result in excessive radial deviation, especially if FCU is also denervated and is therefore no longer favored.[2]

### Thumb and Finger Extension

Thumb extension is approached with PL rerouted subcutaneously to EPL.[30] The EPL is typically transected proximal to the extensor retinaculum and rerouted palmarly (often through the first dorsal compartment) to create a direct line of pull with the PL. Finger extension is then addressed with FCR transfer.[29] FCR is transected at the level of the wrist crease and either routed around the radial border of the forearm or through the interosseous membrane. It is then sutured end to side to each of the EDC tendons. A potential problem with this more conventional reconstruction is the utilization of all wrist flexors in the situation whereby the FCU

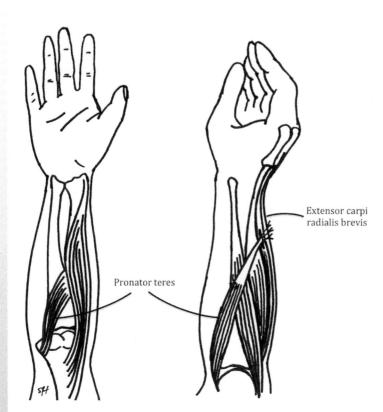

**Fig. 6.** PT to ECRB transfer to restore wrist extension. PT is released from its insertion and brought subcutaneously around the radial border of the forearm, superficial to the BR and ECRL tendons and joined to ECRB in an end-to-side fashion.

Extensor carpi radialis brevis

Pronator teres

is not functional. Usually finger flexors can balance the wrist, but it may lead to other problems with functional training and needs to be considered. An alternative to address both thumb and finger extension is FDS transfer.[29] The index and ring-finger FDS tendons are transected distally, freed, and brought dorsally through the interosseous membrane, proximal to pronator quadratus. The index FDS tendon is sutured into EPL and EIP, while the ring FDS tendon is joined to all EDC tendons. The junction of theses tendons is made proximal to the wrist extensor retinaculum. It should be noted that there have been rehabilitation issues with making extensors from flexors, and therefore, the other options discussed above may be preferable.

### Thumb Adduction

Thumb adduction is addressed with a split FDS tendon transfer.[1,12] The FDS to the middle finger is split, with one-half being brought superficial to adductor pollicis to the insertion of APB, providing thumb adduction to re-create key pinch as well as restoring thumb opposition. Again, if needed, thumb MP fusion can increase pinch power.[1] The other half of the middle-finger FDS is then split in half, with the slips being brought ulnarly and inserted on the A2 pulleys of the ring and small finger, improving coordinated MP and IP flexion.

### Finger Flexion

Flexion of the ring and small fingers can easily be restored by side-to-side suturing of these ulnar innervated MTUs to the FDP tendons of the index and long fingers in the forearm, where the resultant scarring will not be as detrimental (**Fig. 7**).[31]

With FDS used to restore thumb and finger extension as well as key grip and opposition as above, there are the potential complications of weak grip and the formation of swan-neck deformities. As the swan-neck deformities tend to occur late and unpredictably, they are generally not addressed prophylactically. If they do occur, PIPJ arthrodesis or tenodesis can be used as salvage operations.[1]

### HIGH MEDIAN-RADIAL NERVE PALSY

Anatomic deficits
- Loss of all wrist MTUs except FCU, all extrinsic finger extensors and flexors (except ulnar FDP), thenar musculature except adductor pollicis, and deep portion of FPB

Reconstructive goals
- Thumb opposition, mass action grip, and digit extension

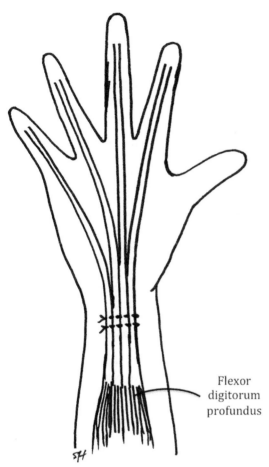

Fig. 7. Side-to-side suturing of FDP tendons in the forearm, allowing mass finger flexion when either the median or the ulnar half of FDP remains innervated.

Available MTUs

- FCU after wrist arthrodesis, ulnar FDP, hypothenar muscles

The high median-radial nerve palsy results in severe deficits and usually necessitates multiple reconstructive surgeries. Traditionally this pattern has had poor outcomes, owing to significant deficits of palmar sensibility combined with loss of all extrinsic finger flexors and extensors and all wrist flexors and extensors with the exception of FCU, leaving few tendons as potential donors.[1] Reconstructive goals are to obtain the most basic of functions, including thumb opposition and mass action grip and digit extension. Because all wrist MTUs are lost except the FCU, radiocarpal arthrodesis is recommended. FCU is then available for transfer to restore digit extension.[16]

## Thumb Opposition

Thumb opposition can be restored using the abductor digiti minimi (ADM) to APB transfer,

also known as the Huber opponensplasty.[32] The ADM is released from its distal insertion and freed proximally, leaving its origin from the pisiform partially intact (**Fig. 8**). It is then turned over like a page in a book and routed subcutaneously across the palm and attached to the APB insertion. Again, the line of pull from the pisiform re-creates the native action of APB. This transfer does, however, remove some function from the small finger, the only digit with full sensation along its radial and ulnar borders. As such, some have advocated carpal metacarpal joint arthrodesis to assist opposition as a more useful procedure in this injury pattern.[16]

## Thumb and Finger Extension

The FCU tendon can be released from its insertions and freed well proximal into the forearm. It can then be tunneled subcutaneously around the ulnar border of the forearm, brought superficial to the EDC and EPL tendons obliquely, and then sutured in place at each tendon junction.

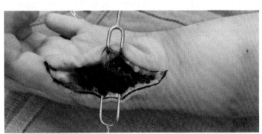

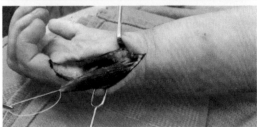

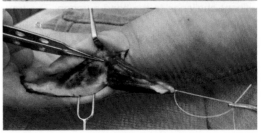

Fig. 8. Intraoperative photographs showing preparation of ADM for transfer to APB to restore thumb opposition. From top to bottom, the muscle is exposed and isolated, and the pisiform origin is partially left intact. It is then turned over like a page in a book and routed subcutaneously across the palm and attached to the APB insertion.

## Thumb and Finger Flexion

To reconstruct finger flexion, the ulnar nerve innervated ring and small finger FDP tendons are sutured side by side into the index and long fingers to allow simple grip in concert.[1] Thumb IPJ flexion is typically restored with FPL tenodesis across the IPJ,[9] with the deep ulnar innervated portion of FBP then driving both MP and IPJ flexion.

## REHABILITATION AND RECOVERY

Because these injuries are rare and each patient's circumstances are unique, there is no place for "cookbook" hand therapy. Everything will need to be individualized and planned ahead of time between therapist and surgeon. Transfers, when possible (and it usually is possible), should be sutured as strong enough to allow early active range of motion to decrease inevitable adhesions.[33] Splinting to avoid overstretching of the transfers also needs to be done in an expert manner and may include finger, wrist, and forearm/elbow joints, depending on the transferred muscles. Later, electrostimulation and biofeedback techniques as well as mirror therapy may be helpful to retrain the transferred muscles to do their new "jobs" correctly.

## CLINICAL RESULTS IN THE LITERATURE

There is little research documenting outcomes of combined peripheral nerve injuries, highlighting the need for further studies. There are some examples of specific procedures used in combined median and ulnar nerve palsy; however, these data are combined with those of single nerve injuries. There have been no outcomes studies on combined medial-radial and ulnar-radial palsies, likely related to the relative infrequency of these injuries.

## SUMMARY

Combined peripheral nerve injuries present a significant challenge to the hand surgeon. The traumatic mechanism of these injuries can result in lacerations to remaining innervated MTUs, significant scar formation, and severe sensory loss. Transfers must be considered on a case-by-case basis and be targeted toward restoring individualized functional goals. With careful planning through identifying anatomic deficits, defining the reconstructive goals, and assessing the available MTUs for transfer, functional improvement can be achieved.

## ACKNOWLEDGMENTS

The authors thank artist, Shelley Hughes, for her illustrations seen in **Figs. 1, 3, 5–7**.

## REFERENCES

1. Omer GE. Tendon transfers for combined traumatic nerve palsies of the forearm and hand. J Hand Surg Br 1992;17(6):603–10.
2. Jones NF, Machado GR. Tendon transfers for radial, median, and ulnar nerve injuries: current surgical techniques. Clin Plast Surg 2011;38(4):621–42.
3. Citron N, Taylor J. Tendon transfer in partially anaesthetic hands. J Hand Surg Br 1987;12(1):14–8.
4. Omer GE Jr. Reconstruction of a balanced thumb through tendon transfers. Clin Orthop Relat Res 1985;(195):104–16.
5. Boyd KU, Nimigan AS, Mackinnon SE. Nerve reconstruction in the hand and upper extremity. Clin Plast Surg 2011;38(4):643–60.
6. Brown JM, Mackinnon SE. Nerve transfers in the forearm and hand. Hand Clin 2008;24(4):319–40, v.
7. Giuffre JL, Bishop AT, Spinner RJ, et al. The best of tendon and nerve transfers in the upper extremity. Plast Reconstr Surg 2015;135(3):617e–30e.
8. Ratner JA, Peljovich A, Kozin SH. Update on tendon transfers for peripheral nerve injuries. J Hand Surg Am 2010;35(8):1371–81.
9. Sammer DM, Chung KC. Tendon transfers: part II. Transfers for ulnar nerve palsy and median nerve palsy. Plast Reconstr Surg 2009;124(3):212e–21e.
10. Seiler JG 3rd, Desai MJ, Payne SH. Tendon transfers for radial, median, and ulnar nerve palsy. J Am Acad Orthop Surg 2013;21(11):675–84.
11. Robinson D, Aghasi MK, Halperin N. Restoration of pinch in ulnar nerve palsy by transfer of split extensor digiti minimi and extensor indicis. J Hand Surg Br 1992;17(6):622–4.
12. Littler JW. Tendon transfers and arthrodeses in combined median and ulnar nerve paralysis. J Bone Joint Surg Am 1949;31A(2):225–34.
13. Smith RJ. Extensor carpi radialis brevis tendon transfer for thumb adduction–a study of power pinch. J Hand Surg Am 1983;8(1):4–15.
14. Omer GE Jr. Tendon transfers in combined nerve lesions. Orthop Clin North Am 1974;5(2):377–87.
15. Van Heest A, Hanson D, Lee J, et al. Split flexor pollicus longus tendon transfer for stabilization of the thumb interphalangeal joint: a cadaveric and clinical study. J Hand Surg Am 1999;24(6):1303–10.
16. Omer GE Jr. Evaluation and reconstruction of the forearm and hand after acute traumatic peripheral nerve injuries. J Bone Joint Surg Am 1968;50(7):1454–78.
17. Burkhalter W, Christensen RC, Brown P. Extensor indicis proprius opponensplasty. J Bone Joint Surg Am 1973;55(4):725–32.
18. Bunnell S. Opposition of the thumb. J Bone Joint Surg Am 1938;20:269–84.
19. Camitz H. Ueber die Behandlung der Opposition-Slahmung. Acta Chir Scand 1929;65:77–81.

20. Littler JW, Li CS. Primary restoration of thumb opposition with median nerve decompression. Plast Reconstr Surg 1967;39(1):74–5.

21. Schneider LH. Opponensplasty using the extensor digiti minimi. J Bone Joint Surg Am 1969;51(7): 1297–302.

22. Phalen GS, Miller RC. The transfer of wrist extensor muscles to restore or reinforce flexion power of the fingers and opposition of the thumb. J Bone Joint Surg Am 1947;29(4):993–7.

23. Curtis RM. Opposition of the thumb. Orthop Clin North Am 1974;5(2):305–21.

24. Cooney WP, Linscheid RL, An KN. Opposition of the thumb: an anatomic and biomechanical study of tendon transfers. J Hand Surg Am 1984;9(6): 777–86.

25. Brand PW. Tendon grafting: illustrated by a new operation for intrinsic paralysis of the fingers. J Bone Joint Surg Br 1961;43:444–53.

26. Brand PW. Tendon transfers for median and ulnar nerve paralysis. Orthop Clin North Am 1970;1(2): 447–54.

27. Parkes A. Paralytic claw fingers–a graft tenodesis operation. Hand 1973;5(3):192–9.

28. Zancolli EA. Claw-hand caused by paralysis of the intrinsic muscles: a simple surgical procedure for its correction. J Bone Joint Surg Am 1957;39A(5): 1076–80.

29. Boyes JH. Tendon transfers for radial palsy. Bull Hosp Joint Dis 1960;21:97–105.

30. Burkhalter WE. Early tendon transfer in upper extremity peripheral nerve injury. Clin Orthop Relat Res 1974;(104):68–79.

31. White WL. Restoration of function and balance of the wrist and hand by tendon transfers. Surg Clin North Am 1960;40:427–59.

32. Littler JW, Cooley SG. Opposition of the thumb and its restoration by abductor digiti quinti transfer. J Bone Joint Surg Am 1963;45:1389–96.

33. Sultana SS, MacDermid JC, Grewal R, et al. The effectiveness of early mobilization after tendon transfers in the hand: a systematic review. J Hand Ther 2013;26(1):1–20 [quiz: 21].

# Tendon Transfers for Tetraplegia

Michael S. Bednar, MD

## KEYWORDS

- Tetraplegia • Quadriplegia • Cervical spinal cord injury • Tendon transfer • Rehabilitation

## KEY POINTS

- It is estimated that 65% to 75% of patients with cervical spinal cord injuries could benefit from upper extremity tendon transfer surgery.
- The goals of surgery are to restore elbow extension, as well as hand pinch, grasp, and release.
- Patients who have defined goals, actively participate in therapy, and understand expected outcomes appear to have the highest satisfaction following tendon transfer procedures.

It is estimated that in the United States there are 12,500 new cases of spinal cord injury each year and 276,000 people currently living with a spinal cord injury. Men constitute 80% of spinal cord injury victims. Approximately 45% of spinal cord injuries result in incomplete tetraplegia and 14% in complete tetraplegia. The lifetime cost of a patient with C5–8 tetraplegia injured at age 25 is estimated at $3,452,781. It is estimated that a person who sustains a C5–8 cervical spinal cord injury at age 20 will live 40 years with his or her injury.[1]

Patients with tetraplegia face many physical, functional, and psychological limitations. Physically, they have difficulty controlling the arm in space and limited or absent grip and pinch strength. Functionally, there is a decrease in mobility, activity of daily living (ADL) performance, and independence with work tasks. The appearance of the hand and patient confidence in social interactions are additional psychological challenges. When patients are asked what function they would most like restored, more patients desired hand function (75%) than bowel and bladder use (13%), walking (8%), and sexual performance (3%).[2]

The goals of surgical reconstruction of the upper limb in tetraplegia are to increase independence and upper extremity function through elbow control for reaching overhead, weight shifting, and transfer; restoration of hand function to allow lateral pinch for self-catheterization, dressing, and ADLs; and grasp and release for feeding and ADLs. Although it is estimated that approximately 65% to 75% of cervical spinal cord patients would benefit from upper extremity surgery to improve on these functional limitations, fewer than 400 of these surgeries are performed per year.[3,4] In other words, only 14% of patients who are surgical candidates actually have tendon transfer procedures.[5] A variety of reasons have been proposed to explain why so few patients have surgery, including a lack of communication among rehabilitation specialists, physiatrists, and surgeons; poor access to care; and poor knowledge that such procedures are possible. A lack of coordinated cross-specialty collaboration appears to be the greatest barrier to appropriate use of upper extremity reconstruction in patients with cervical spinal cord injury.[5]

## CERVICAL SPINE INJURY AND CLASSIFICATION

Spinal cord injuries are classified using the American Spinal Injury Association (ASIA) impairment scale (**Table 1**),[6] which grades the degree of spinal

The author is a consultant for Zimmer Biomet.

Division of Hand Surgery, Department of Orthopaedic Surgery and Rehabilitation, Stritch School of Medicine, Loyola University, 1700 Maguire Building, 2160 South First Avenue, Maywood, IL 60153, USA

*E-mail address:* mbednar@lumc.edu

**Table 1**
**American Spinal Injury Association (ASIA) impairment scale**

| ASIA Grade | Patient Function |
|---|---|
| A | Complete, no sensory or motor preserved distal to injury, no sacral preservation |
| B | Incomplete sensory, sensory preserved below injury level, including sacral, no motor preservation |
| C | Motor incomplete, more than half of the key muscle functions below level of injury have grade <3 strength |
| D | Motor incomplete, at least half of motor below level grade >3 strength |
| E | Normal |

**Table 3**
**International Classification for Surgery of the Hand in Tetraplegia**

| Class | Description |
|---|---|
| 0 | No functioning muscles |
| 1 | Brachioradialis |
| 2 | Extensor carpi radial longus |
| 3 | Extensor carpi radial brevis |
| 4 | Pronator teres |
| 5 | Flexor carpi radialis |
| 6 | Extensor digitorum communis |
| 7 | Thumb extensors |
| 8 | Partial finger flexors |
| 9 | All but intrinsics |
| X | Exceptions |

The ICSHT determines the number of muscles present below the elbow with at least grade 4 strength. The muscles are listed in the order in which recovery is expected in complete tetraplegia.

cord injury from A to E and as complete or incomplete based on the lowest functioning cord segment. Manual motor testing graded 0 to 5 is based on the British Medical Research Scale (**Table 2**).[7] A motor score of 0 to 100 is given based on the sum of the motor grades in 5 key upper and lower extremity functions bilaterally. The total upper extremity score is 0 to 50 and based on elbow flexion, wrist extension, elbow extension, finger flexion, and finger abduction.

Although the ASIA classification is widely used to categorize patients with tetraplegia, the levels are too broad to make decisions about reconstructive procedures of the upper extremities. The International Classification for Surgery of the Hand in Tetraplegia (ICSHT) was developed to evaluate the upper extremity and formulate a treatment plan for patients with tetraplegia (**Table 3**).

## PATIENT EVALUATION

A thorough history begins with age, preexisting conditions, and medications. Patients should be asked about past and present opioid use. The history of the spinal cord injury includes date of injury, method of injury, spinal cord injury level, other associated injuries, and surgical history. The patient's functional goals should be discussed to determine what activities the patient would like to regain. In evaluating the upper extremities, the examiner should identify which arm is now the dominant extremity. All muscles of the upper extremity are graded with manual motor testing. Joints are placed through active and passive range of motion. Contractures or spasticity are noted. Patients are examined for concomitant brachial plexus injuries.

The brachioradialis (BR) is palpated with the elbow flexed at 90° and the forearm in neutral rotation while active elbow flexion is resisted with a forced applied to the distal forearm. The muscle is too weak to transfer if the muscle belly can easily be displaced anteriorly and posteriorly. It also is important to determine if both the extensor carpi radialis longus (ECRL) and brevis (ECRB) are functioning. Both are usually intact if the wrist extension strength is 5/5 and there is a groove or depression distal to the lateral epicondyle with strength testing (Bean sign).[8] Allieu and colleagues[9] stated that if the pronator teres (PT) is

**Table 2**
**British Medical Research Scale manual motor testing**

| Grade | Function |
|---|---|
| 5 | Full motion against gravity and full resistance |
| 4 | Full motion against gravity and moderate resistance |
| 3 | Full motion against gravity only |
| 2 | Full motion with gravity eliminated |
| 1 | Trace motion/palpable or visible contraction |
| 0 | No contraction/paralysis |

at least 4/5 then it can be assumed that both ECRL and ECRB are functioning. If the ECRL alone is functioning, the wrist radially deviates with extension, because it inserts on the second metacarpal and wrist extension can easily be overcome when the examiner pushes the wrist into flexion with one finger.

## TREATMENT PRINCIPLES

Early treatment of the upper limb begins during inpatient rehabilitation by maintaining passive range of motion, preventing injury/overstretch of the thumb metacarpophalangeal joint, increasing functional use of hands, and maximizing wrist and elbow strength and finger tenodesis. It is important to use adaptive equipment to increase use of hands, improve independence, and prevent development of destructive patterns that would lead to tendon and ligament incompetence. The final part of early treatment is to educate patients and their families on surgical procedures to increase upper extremity function.

When patients are identified as surgical candidates, they should be evaluated early by a team consisting of the patient, caregivers, physiatrist, occupational therapist, nurse, social worker, and hand surgeon. Once a patient's ICSHT level is known and functional goals are established, the team decides whether they think the patient is a good surgical candidate. A good surgical candidate has functional goals, is motivated, understands benefits and limitations of surgery, demonstrates emotional and psychological stability/adjustment to disability, and is committed to the postoperative rehabilitation process. Patients should have cervical spine injury levels C5–8 and ICSHT 1 or better. The timing of when to perform the surgery is a balance between stabilization of the patient's neurologic, emotional, and social recovery from the spinal cord injury and undertaking surgery, which will temporarily decrease a patient's independence during the rehabilitation process. In the United States, surgery is usually delayed for approximately a year after injury to allow the patient to accept the injury and maximize his or her gains with therapy. Because there is often a lag between postinjury rehabilitation and surgery, it is usually necessary to have patients seen for a limited number of therapy sessions before any surgical procedures. This will address joint contractures, muscle weakness, and trunk conditioning. Patients and their caretakers need to practice transfers with a cast on the arm or without using the involved arm. Electric wheelchair controls need to be moved to the nonoperative side.

## SURGICAL MANAGEMENT

The mainstay of tetraplegic upper extremity surgery is tendon transfers. Donor muscles must be expendable and have adequate strength and excursion. If the patient's needs exceed the number of donor muscles, other procedures, such as tenodesis and arthrodesis, may be used.

Contraindications to surgery include active infections, open wounds, pressure sores, poor soft tissue bed, bony instability or laxity, painful paresthesias, medical instability, spasticity, and joint contractures.

## ELBOW EXTENSION RECONSTRUCTION

Approximately 75% patients with tetraplegia lose elbow extension. Elbow extension improves mobility in bed, independence with transfers, safety with driving, balance with sitting, weight shifting, overhead reach, and manual wheelchair use. It functions as an antagonist to the brachioradialis, improving the ability of this muscle to function after transfer. The 2 methods to improve elbow extension are the posterior deltoid–to-triceps transfer and the biceps-to-triceps transfer.

The posterior deltoid–to-triceps transfer is done with a lateral incision over the deltoid to elevate the posterior one-third to one-half of the deltoid from humeral insertion. Splitting the deltoid too far proximally can injure the axillary nerve. The radial nerve is behind the lateral head of the triceps and brachialis. The deltoid insertion is a broad, short tendon, which makes a secure tendon transfer difficult. The deltoid insertion may be elevated with a bony segment of the humerus to improve the quality of the tendon for transfer. If the deltoid insertion is elevated without bone, the transfer is augmented with a tibialis anterior free tendon graft, fascia lata, or Dacron tape. The central third of the triceps tendon is elevated from the olecranon in a distal to proximal direction. The proximal dissection ends approximately 1 to 2 cm from the musculotendinous junctions of the triceps. The central third of the triceps is woven through the deltoid tendon and sutured with 2-0 nonabsorbable sutures. The supplemental tendon graft or synthetic tape is woven through the triceps to reinforce this transfer. Tension is set so that the patient has no more than 45° of passive elbow flexion following the procedure. The tendons of the triceps that remain medially and laterally distal are sutured together.

The poor tendon quality of the posterior deltoid tendon makes this weave prone to elongation. Arm positioning is crucial to success of the procedure.[10] Postoperatively, the patient is placed into a long-arm splint in extension, which is removed at postoperative day 3 to 5 and changed to a hinged elbow brace. This is locked into full extension for 4 weeks and worn continuously for 11 weeks. Beginning the fifth postoperative week, elbow extension in the hinged brace is increased at 15° per week. The patient is cautioned to not allow arm to cross midline for 11 weeks. When in a wheelchair, the arm is placed in a trough and abduction bar to keep the arm abducted. In bed, the shoulder should be abducted 30° with an abduction pillow.

Wangdell and Fridén[11] reported outcomes at 6 months and 1 year from surgery. Improvement was seen in all activities, especially propelling a wheelchair and reaching out. No patient rated any goals lower than before surgery.

When performing a biceps-to-triceps transfer, a patient must have intact brachialis and supinator to flex and supinate postoperatively.[12] An anterior incision is made over the distal half of the medial side of the biceps and then curved over the antecubital fossa to harvest the biceps tendon. The lacertus fibrosis is released and the biceps tendon is transected within 1 cm of its insertion. The biceps muscle is freed of fascial attachments proximally until the most distal motor branches from the musculocutaneous nerve are seen entering the muscle. A posterior incision is made beginning 6 cm proximal to the olecranon in the midline, curving laterally around the olecranon and onto the subcutaneous border of the ulna. The biceps tendon is passed subcutaneously along the medial side to avoid compression of radial nerve. It is necessary to widely dissect the facial attachment between the anterior and posterior compartments of the arm to allow the biceps muscle belly to freely pass through this space. The triceps tendon is split over the tip of the olecranon. A 10-mm drill is passed through the proximal cortex of the olecranon, aiming toward but not perforating the lateral cortex of the olecranon. Two, number 2 nonabsorbable, braided sutures of different colors are placed in a Krakow fashion 90° to each other. The biceps tendon is woven twice through the triceps tendon, with the second weave exiting at the triceps tendon split where the olecranon drill hole was made. Two large Keith needles are then placed into the large olecranon hole and drilled through the lateral cortex of the olecranon. Sutures of different colors are placed in the eye of each Keith needle and pulled through the lateral cortex. Tension on the sutures pulls the tendon into the olecranon drill hole. Tension is set so that the patient has no more than 45° of passive elbow flexion following the procedure. The transfer is reinforced with 2 to 0 nonabsorbable sutures between the biceps and triceps tendons. The postoperative course is the same as for the deltoid to triceps with the exception that the precautions against the arm crossing the midline do not pertain. The patient learns to activate the transfer by asking the patient to supinate the forearm.

Mulcahey and colleagues[13] compared 8 deltoid transfers with 8 biceps transfers for triceps extension, and at 24-month follow-up 7 of 8 biceps transfers were grade 3 or better and 1 of 8 deltoid transfers was grade 3. There was considerable but subclinical loss of elbow flexion torque (biceps 47%, deltoid 32%).

## HAND RECONSTRUCTION

The choice of which procedures are available for hand reconstruction are dependent on what muscles are functioning and expendable. If active extension of the wrist is not present, it needs to be the first priority to improve hand function. Arthrodesis of the wrist in general should be avoided because the patient will lose the ability to use the tenodesis effect on tendons for motion.[14]

It is helpful to use the ICSHT to evaluate possible surgeries to restore hand function.

Group 0 has no motors intact below the elbow and therefore has no muscles available for transfer to improve hand function. Static splints and orthoses can be used to assist in function.

In group 1, transfer of the BR to the ECRB will provide active wrist extension. This motor allows for the use of a dynamic orthosis.[15]

In the Moberg procedure, the BR is transferred to the ECRB and the flexor pollicis longus (FPL) is tenodesed to the ulnar side of the distal radius with the goal of pulling the thumb into lateral pinch when the wrist is actively extended. As originally described, the interphalangeal joint of the thumb is pinned for more stable pinch. If the metacarpophalangeal joint is very flexible, the extensor pollicis longus (EPL) and extensor pollicis brevis (EPB) are tenodesed to the thumb metacarpal to stabilize the joint against excessive flexion during pinch. Hentz and colleagues[3] showed good results in 18 limbs (55%) with improved postoperative performance of functional activities (self-care, communication, and mobility). Three of 11 patients required revision to tighten FPL tenodesis, further stabilize the metacarpophalangeal (MP) joint, or to replace extruded interphalangeal (IP) joint pins. Poor results were seen in 5 patients, but none asked for reversal of surgery and did not think function was worsened from procedure.

In group 2, the BR and ECRL are functioning. The ECRL is retained for active wrist extension.

The BR is transferred to the FPL to provide active pinch. The IP joint of the thumb is stabilized with a screw or wire. If active thumb extension is not present, the EPL and EPB tendons are tenodesed to the metacarpal. Waters and colleagues[16] reviewed 15 patients (16 thumbs) with functional improvement seen in 15 hands.[17] Eighty percent could name at least 4 activities of daily living now possible after surgery. With the elbow flexed to 90° and the wrist extended there was an average of 3.9 pounds of lateral pinch strength, 4 pounds with wrist neutral and 2.3 pounds with the wrist flexed to 30°. There was a direct correlation between pinch strength and amount of triceps and wrist extensor strength.

Group 3 has BR, ECRL, and ECRB function. There is controversy concerning whether hand reconstruction should be for pinch and grasp or only pinch. When reconstructing to restore pinch and grasp, the BR is transferred to the FPL and the ECRL is transferred to the flexor digitorum profundus (FDP). The ECRB is left to provide centralized wrist extension. Proponents of reconstructing pinch alone believe that the ECRB may be too weak to provide wrist extension against the BR and ECRL, whose transferred vectors now make them wrist flexors. Loss of active wrist extension causes loss of hand tenodesis and worsening of hand function. Proponents of reconstructing pinch and grasp recommend transferring the ECRB to the FDP and leaving the stronger ECRL for active wrist extension. Grasp may not be as strong and wrist extension may be more radially deviated than in a group 4 patient, but these surgeons believe the restoration of grasp improves the patient's function.

In group 4, BR, ECRL, ECRB, and PT are functioning. The goals of upper limb reconstruction in these patients are pinch, grasp, and release. The functions needed in this group are finger extension, thumb extension, intrinsic function, finger and thumb flexion, and thumb carpometacarpal (CMC) stability. This is typically accomplished in 2 stages but some investigators are reporting good results with a 1-stage operation.[18]

Stage 1 is the extensor phase, where thumb and finger extension is accomplished through tenodesis with optional intrinsic balancing.[15] Extensor digitorum comminus (EDC) tenodesis is accomplished by suturing the tendons to achieve a reverse cascade effect, with the index finger being the most flexed to allow proper position for pinch and the small finger being the least flexed to keep it out of the way during grasp. An ulnarly based U-shaped trough is made on the dorsoradial side of the distal radius proximal to the Lister tubercle. The EDC tendons are passed under this bony peninsula to shorten their excursion and tenodese

them to the bone. Tension is set to attain full-finger MP extension with the wrist at neutral. In general, tenodesis operations stretch with time. By the end of 3 months of therapy, full-finger MP extension usually occurs with the wrist in 30° of flexion.

If there is excessive clawing of the digits after the EDC tenodesis, an intrinsic tenodesis is done during the extensor phase (see Hand Intrinsic Balancing).

Thumb extension is produced by EPL tenodesis to extend the MP joint and FPL split tenodesis to maintain the IP joint in extension. The FPL is split over the proximal phalanx and the radial half is detached from the distal phalanx. It is retracted proximally out of the oblique pulley and woven into the EPL over the proximal portion of the proximal phalanx. When tension is applied to the FPL, the force is equalized palmarly and dorsally at the IP joint and the FPL now produces active flexion at the MP joint.[8] For the EPL tenodesis, the EPL is transected at its musculotendinous junction. The EPL tendon is left in the third dorsal compartment. The retinaculum is removed over the tendon distal to the Lister tubercle. The proximal end is brought distal to the extensor retinaculum and is sutured to the tendon distal to the Lister tubercle, tensioned to allow thumb extension with the wrist neutral.

Thumb stability, position, and control can be attained with either an opponensplasty or a CMC arthrodesis. In the opponensplasty, either the PT or BR is transferred to the tendon of the flexor digitorum superficialis (FDS) ring in the forearm. The tendon is transected proximal to its decussation, retracted into the palm, and wrapped around the palmar fascial to act as a pulley. The distal end of the tendon is woven to the tendon of the abductor pollicis brevis. With thumb CMC arthrodesis, the thumb is pre-positioned for lateral pinch. The general parameters of the fusion are 20° to 25° extension, 40° to 45° abduction, and slight pronation.

Following the procedure, the patient is placed into a dorsal blocking splint in 30° wrist extension, 30° MCP flexion, 20° to 30° IP flexion, and thumb position dictated by fusion position. This is worn continuously for 4 weeks. Tenodesis motion is initiated at 4 weeks postoperatively by gently bringing the wrist from extension to flexion. At week 8, the patient may begin strengthening and restoration of full passive motion to prepare for stage 2 surgery.

Stage 2 is the flexor phase, in which the ECRL is transferred to the FDP tendons to restore grasp and the ECRB is retained as the wrist extensor. The BR is transferred to the FPL tendon for pinch. The FDP tendons are first sewn together, reversing the cascade of the digits. The tension of the transfers should be set such that when the wrist is flexed, the fingers and thumb should be fully extended and when the wrist is extended the fingers should be flexed and the thumb pulp resting on the side of the middle phalanx of the index finger. The fingers must flex before the thumb adducts to prevent a thumb in palm deformity.

A dorsal blocking splint with wrist neutral, MPs 60° flexion, IPs slight flexion, and thumb in lateral pinch is worn for approximately 4 weeks. If the tendon weave is done using modified Pulvertaft weave, then the patient is allowed to begin early place and hold exercises, in which the fingers and thumb are passively placed in fist and held by the patient with wrist extension before slowly relaxing into an extended position.[18] Active range of motion is begun at approximately 10 days with pinch and grip, and light functional tasks after 2 weeks. The patient can begin wheelchair propulsion at 4 weeks and functional transfers at weeks 6 to 8.

House and Shannon[15] showed significant improvement in strength and speed for activities of daily living. There were 6 patients with one side undergoing a CMC fusion and the other an opponensplasty. Both methods provided lateral pinch and strong grasp with patient preference divided. The ability to button, tie shoes, dress, and transfer were all improved. Wangdell and Fridén[11] reviewed patient satisfaction and performance of identified activity goals after thumb and finger flexion reconstruction on average 7 years after surgery using BR to FPL and ECRL to FDP transfers and reported improvement in all groups of activities in the Canadian Occupational Performance Measure. The most improvement was observed for eating, but significant improvement was seen in more complex activities, such as housework and leisure activities.

Hamou and colleagues[17] reviewed results in a meta-analysis of pinch strength following reconstruction procedures; adverse outcomes were approximately 40%, which included 35% elbow or thumb contracture, 22% stretching or rupture of repair, 21% loosening of pins at thumb IP joint, and 10% misalignment of pinch. Overall, mean postoperative pinch strength was 2 kg (1 kg for tenodesis, 2 kg with active motor).

Group 5 patients have the addition of flexor carpi radialis, which is usually retained for better wrist control and better finger extension secondary to active wrist flexion. In group 4 patients who have poor release, the PT can be transferred to the flexor carpi radialis (FCR) to improve finger extension. An adduction-opponensplasty can be performed using the BR, PT, or flexor carpi ulnaris (FCU) in groups 7 and 8 via the FDS tendon graft.

## HAND INTRINSIC BALANCING

The intrinsics provide smooth grasp and release when coupled with extrinsic procedures so as to avoid early finger roll-up when trying to grasp objects. Indications for surgery are proximal interphalangeal joint flexion deformity (from FDS spasticity or central slip incompetence), central slip deficits, and metacarpophalangeal joint hyperextension. Intrinsic tenodesis is performed by passing a free tendon graft dorsal to the index metacarpal neck and a second free tendon graft is placed dorsal to the ring finger metacarpal neck.[15] The graft is passed palmar to the deep transverse intermetacarpal ligament by inserting a tendon passer along the lumbrical canal from distally to proximally. The distal ends of the tendon graft are sewn to the radial lateral bands. If the central slips are deficient, the tendon graft is sewn distally to the insertion of the central slip on the middle phalanx. As the extrinsic tendon pulls the finger into extension, the proximal interphalangeal (PIP) joint will extend through a tenodesis effect. This is performed at the same time and stage as extensor communis tenodesis and is most beneficial with central slip deficits.

The Zancolli[19] lasso procedure releases the FDS tendon distally and turns it back on itself around the A1 pulley to create dynamic MP joint flexion when the wrist is extended. This is done in the flexor stage of the reconstruction and is especially useful for significant clawing (MP hyperextension) and PIP flexion deformity from FDS spasticity. This will move the flexion force from the PIP joint to the MP joint.[20]

The third procedure is the modified Stiles-Bunnell procedure, in which the middle finger FDS tendon is taken off its insertion distally, divided into multiple slips, rerouted along the path of the lumbricals, volar to the deep transverse metacarpal ligament, and attached to the lateral band and central slip.[21,22]

McCarthy and colleagues[20] reviewed 183 hand reconstructions and compared extrinsic reconstructions with and without in intrinsic balancing. They found that the patients with intrinsic balancing had increased grip strength (13–26 N) over those without. There were no differences between the free tendon graft tenodesis and the lasso procedure and no statistical difference for scores of activities of daily living for all patients.

## LONG-TERM OUTCOMES

Wuolle and colleagues[23] found 77% of patients report positive life impact and 70% were satisfied with surgery for their tetraplegia. Mohammed and colleagues[8] showed 70% good or excellent results and 84% reported that surgery improved their quality of life. Patients report that surgeries do not always improve independence but do provide increased spontaneity, speed, and ease of picking up objects and other specific tasks.

Hamou and colleagues[17] reported a positive risk-benefit ratio of greater than 2 with significant improvement in upper limb function versus adverse outcomes. Dunn and colleagues[24] looked at changes in hand strength over time after tenodesis or active tendon transfer surgery. They previously reported that patients maintained or improved pinch and grip strength during the 12 to 18 years following surgery, and re-reviewed 19 of these patients 11 years later.[25] They found that the active key pinch strength decreased 14% on the right and 1% on the left; whereas in the tenodesis group there was a decrease of 40% on the right and 51% on the left. The mean pinch strength was 11.5 N in the tenodesis group and 32.9 N in the active transfers group. There was also no significant change in grip strength between the 2 time measurements but the active group strength decreased by 5% to 8% and the tenodesis group increased by 32% to 70%. The mean grip for active transfers was 59 N and 23 N for the tenodesis group. Both pinch and grip strength were increased triple and double the amounts, respectively, in the active group compared with the tenodesis group. Most patients reported little change in functioning over the 11 years, but 50% reported decline in ability to propel their wheelchair and approximately 35% reported decline in their ability to raise themselves from the seat.

## SUMMARY

Tendon transfers for reconstruction of the upper limb in tetraplegia is an underused resource for this population. Although the long-term outcomes of these procedures are good, few patients eligible for these procedures actually have them performed. Continued education of patients with tetraplegia, their caregivers, and the rehabilitation community will hopefully increase utilization of these effective tendon transfer procedures.

## REFERENCES

1. Spinal cord injury fact and figures at a glance. Birmingham (AL): National Spinal Cord Injury Statistical Center; 2014.
2. Hanson RW, Franklin MR. Sexual loss in relation to other functional losses for spinal cord injured males. Arch Phys Med Rehabil 1976;57:291–3.
3. Hentz VR, Brown M, Keoshian LA. Upper limb reconstruction in quadriplegia: functional assessment and proposed treatment modifications. J Hand Surg Am 1983;8:119–31.
4. Moberg E. Surgical treatment for absent single-hand grip and elbow extension in quadriplegia. Principles and preliminary experience. J Bone Joint Surg Am 1975;57:196–206.
5. Curtin CM, Gater DR, Chung KC. Upper extremity reconstruction in the tetraplegic population, a national epidemiologic study. J Hand Surg Am 2005;30:94–9.
6. Association ASI. International standards for neurological classification of spinal cord injury. 2014.
7. Compston A. Aids to the investigation of peripheral nerve injuries. Medical Research Council: Nerve Injuries Research Committee. His Majesty's Stationery Office: 1942; pp. 48 (iii) and 74 figures and 7 diagrams; with aids to the examination of the peripheral nervous system. By Michael O'Brien for the Guarantors of Brain. Saunders Elsevier: 2010; pp. [8] 64 and 94 Figures. Brain 2010;133: 2838–44.
8. Mohammed KD, Rothwell AG, Sinclair SW, et al. Upper-limb surgery for tetraplegia. J Bone Joint Surg Br 1992;74:873–9.
9. Allieu Y, Coulet B, Chammas M. Functional surgery of the upper limb in high-level tetraplegia: part I. Tech Hand Up Extrem Surg 2000;4: 50–63.
10. Fridén J, Ejeskär A, Dahlgren A, et al. Protection of the deltoid to triceps tendon transfer repair sites. J Hand Surg Am 2000;25:144–9.
11. Wangdell J, Fridén J. Activity gains after reconstructions of elbow extension in patients with tetraplegia. J Hand Surg Am 2012;37:1003–10.
12. Kuz JE, Van Heest AE, House JH. Biceps-to-triceps transfer in tetraplegic patients: report of the medial routing technique and follow-up of three cases. J Hand Surg Am 1999;24:161–72.
13. Mulcahey MJ, Lutz C, Kozin SH, et al. Prospective evaluation of biceps to triceps and deltoid to triceps for elbow extension in tetraplegia. J Hand Surg Am 2003;28:964–71.
14. Lamb DW, Chan KM. Surgical reconstruction of the upper limb in traumatic tetraplegia. A review of 41 patients. J Bone Joint Surg Br 1983;65: 291–8.
15. House JH, Shannon MA. Restoration of strong grasp and lateral pinch in tetraplegia: a comparison of two methods of thumb control in each patient. J Hand Surg Am 1985;10:22–9.
16. Waters R, Moore KR, Graboff SR, et al. Brachioradialis to flexor pollicis longus tendon transfer for active lateral pinch in the tetraplegic. J Hand Surg Am 1985;10:385–91.
17. Hamou C, Shah NR, DiPonio L, et al. Pinch and elbow extension restoration in people with

tetraplegia: a systematic review of the literature. J Hand Surg Am 2009;34:692–9.

18. Reinholdt C, Fridén J. Outcomes of single-stage grip-release reconstruction in tetraplegia. J Hand Surg Am 2013;38:1137–44.

19. Zancolli E. Structural and dynamic bases of hand surgery. 2nd edition. Philadelphia: JB Lippincott; 1979.

20. McCarthy CK, House JH, Van Heest A, et al. Intrinsic balancing in reconstruction of the tetraplegic hand. J Hand Surg Am 1997;22:596–604.

21. Sammer DM, Chung KC. Tendon transfers: part II. Transfers for ulnar nerve palsy and median nerve palsy. Plast Reconstr Surg 2009;124:212e–21e.

22. Bunnell S. Surgery of the intrinsic muscles of the hand other than those producing opposition of the thumb. J Bone Joint Surg 1942;XXIV:1–31.

23. Wuolle KS, Bryden AM, Peckham PH, et al. Satisfaction with upper-extremity surgery in individuals with tetraplegia. Arch Phys Med Rehabil 2003; 84:1145–9.

24. Dunn JA, Rothwell AG, Mohammed KD, et al. The effects of aging on upper limb tendon transfers in patients with tetraplegia. J Hand Surg Am 2014;39: 317–23.

25. Rothwell AG, Sinnott KA, Mohammed KD, et al. Upper limb surgery for tetraplegia: a 10-year re-review of hand function. J Hand Surg Am 2003;28:489–97.

# Free Flap Functional Muscle Transfers

Ryan M. Garcia, MD[a],*, David S. Ruch, MD[b]

## KEYWORDS

- Free • Functional • Muscle • Flap • Transfer

## KEY POINTS

- Free functional muscle transfers remain a powerful upper extremity reconstructive option when other local transfers are unavailable.
- Selection of the donor motor nerve remains challenging, particularly following brachial plexus injuries.
- The gracilis muscle is most commonly used as the donor given its functional capacity, ease of harvest, and disguised donor site.
- Variable outcomes have been reported following free functional muscle transfers that are related to donor motor nerve availability and reinnervation.

## INTRODUCTION

Upper extremity functional muscle loss secondary to brachial plexus injuries, ischemic muscle loss, traumatic injuries, oncologic resections, or congenital absences can be life altering and may severely limit a patient's ability to perform activities of daily living. More commonly, upper extremity functional losses are reconstructed with local muscle and tendon transfers.[1] Alternatively, upper extremity functional losses also can be treated by performing a neurotization procedure that entails using some or all fascicles of an intact donor motor nerve and transferring the afferent signal to a distal recipient nerve with a viable, available muscle.[2] Less commonly, patients who are not candidates for a tendon, local pedicled muscle, or nerve transfer may be considered for a functional free muscle transfer to restore elbow flexion, finger and wrist flexion, and/or finger and wrist extension.

Functional free muscle transfers were first explored in dogs and reported by Tamai and colleagues in 1970.[3] Terzis and colleagues[4] later showed in a rabbit model that only one-fourth of the rectus muscle function was retained after free muscle transfer and replantation. These findings were later challenged in 1986 by Stevanovic and colleagues[5] in a canine study that demonstrated 70% of the transplanted muscle function could be achieved following the free muscle transfer. Regarding upper extremity functional muscle transfers, Manktelow and McKee[6] were the first to report on 2 cases (1 gracilis muscle, 1 pectoralis major muscle) to restore finger flexion after traumatic injuries in what were reported to be excellent outcomes. Ikuta and colleagues[7] shortly thereafter reported a free gracilis muscle transfer to restore elbow flexion in a patient with brachial plexopathy.

## PATIENT SELECTION

Stevanovic and Sharpe[8] provided a number of guidelines for appropriate patient selection before performing a free functional muscle transfer. First, patient motivation must be assessed. Patients need to have an acceptable expectation and need to be compliant with the planned postoperative course, which entails extensive and complex

Disclosures: The authors have no conflicts of interest.
a OrthoCarolina, Division of Hand Surgery, Hand Center, 1915 Randolph Road, 2nd Floor, Charlotte, NC 28207, USA; b Department of Orthopedic Surgery, Duke University Medical Center, 2301 Erwin Road, Durham, NC 27705, USA
* Corresponding author.
E-mail address: ryan.garcia@orthocarolina.com

hand.theclinics.com

physical therapy rehabilitation. These investigators also recommended an age consideration of 45 years or younger for patients considering this complex reconstruction. Despite this arbitrary age consideration, others have reported excellent outcomes in patients much older.[9] Less has been reported on free flap reconstructions in skeletally immature patients[10–12] and the long-term outcomes in this subgroup of patients remains unknown. Although Terzis and Kostopoulos[13] did show improved outcomes in patients younger than 15 years following free muscle transfer for elbow flexion, these patients should be informed on the potential for asymmetrical growth of the transplanted muscle when compared with the growing skeleton, which could lead to future joint contractures and weakened muscle strength. Stevanovic and Sharpe[8] also highlighted that patients with medical comorbidities compromising vascular microcirculation and nerve reinnervation, such as diabetes, peripheral vascular disease, autoimmune diseases, and smoking, should be contraindicated for free functional muscle transfers.

## HIERARCHY OF FUNCTIONAL RESTORATION

The hierarchy of functional restoration for the upper extremity remains elbow flexion,[1] finger flexion, and finger extension allowing patients to improve their ability to perform vital activities of daily living. Ideally, the general tendon transfer principle of using a single muscle to provide a single function applies to free functional muscle transfers. Despite this, when there is a paucity of donor motor nerves to power multiple free functional muscles in a single limb, then a single muscle may be used to accomplish multiple functions. Hattori and colleagues and Doi and colleagues,[14–17] in a series of articles, reported the use of a double free muscle transfer in which 1 muscle was used to provide both elbow flexion and wrist extension while the second muscle transfer was responsible for finger flexion. These investigators reported good-to-excellent outcomes in most patients, which included both children[14] and adults.[15–17] In the series of patients with long-term follow-up, 25 (96%) of 26 patients were determined to have good-to-excellent elbow flexion and 17 (65%) of 26 had good-to-excellent hand prehension capabilities.[16] Most investigators use the British Medical Research Council Grading System to report preoperative and postoperative outcomes and are referenced throughout this article.

## RECIPIENT SITE

Many of the established tendon transfer principles also apply to the use of free functional muscle transfers. These principles include the following: the use of a single muscle/tendon to provide a single function, confirming that the joint involved in the transfer is as supple as possible having maximized passive range of motion capabilities, the muscle should be oriented to provide a straight line of pull to maximize the muscle effect on the joint, an adequate muscle antagonist should be present, optimization of the synergistic effects of distal joints whenever possible, and the soft tissue bed should be adequate to support the muscle while also allowing the tendon to glide. Stevanovic and Sharpe[8] further expand these requirements for free functional muscle transfers to include an adequate donor motor nerve and available vessels for microsurgical anastomosis. The available donor motor nerve should be expendable, have a maximized number of axons, and should be of adequate length (often increased with nerve grafts) to allow a tension-free coaptation.

Additional surgical interventions may be necessary before the free functional muscle transfer. Patients who do not demonstrate adequate passive range of motion may require a joint capsulotomy/capsulectomy and contracture release or extensive tenolysis followed by an extended period of aggressive physical therapy. The soft tissue bed also can be optimized to allow eventual tendon gliding. This may require resection of scar tissue and soft tissue rearrangement procedures before the microsurgical reconstruction.

## DONOR MOTOR NERVES

The donor motor nerves available for neurotization can be challenging, particularly in patients with complete brachial plexus injuries. In contrast, patients who undergo a functional free muscle transfer after a Volkmann contracture, traumatic injury, or oncologic resection often have various local donor motor nerves readily available. When possible, it is preferred to choose the donor nerve with the same or similar function as the anticipated free muscle transfer. In scenarios in which the donor motor nerve is chosen from a very distant site, it is advised that the nerve is established and allowed to mature before the free functional muscle transfer. Terzis and Kostopoulos[13] demonstrated this principle in a large series of patients who underwent free muscle transfers after posttraumatic brachial plexopathies to restore elbow function and hand function.[18] The distant donor motor nerve was chosen, nerve grafts coapted, and tunneled to the "banked" recipient site during the first stage of the reconstruction. The second stage consists of transferring the free functional muscle, which typically occurs 6 to 9 months later depending on the length of the coapted nerve grafts. The first stage ("banking" procedure) allows the chosen donor motor nerve axons to mature through the necessary grafts so as to shorten the time period for muscle reinnervation after the muscle has been transplanted. The most common motor nerves in patients with complete brachial plexopathies to restore elbow flexion included intercostals, spinal accessory, contralateral lateral pectoral, ipsilateral C5, and contralateral C7.[13] Terzis and Kostopoulos[18] found that when the gracilis was chosen as the donor muscle, better outcomes occurred with the spinal accessory nerve; however, these findings were not statistically significant. These investigators also found that if intercostal nerves were used, improved outcomes occurred with the latissimus dorsi muscle when compared with the gracilis muscle. Additionally, 3 intercostals were found to outperform the use of only 2 intercostals. In a later article, these same investigators described the various donor motor nerves chosen to restore finger flexion in patients with brachial plexopathies. Choices for finger flexion included intercostals (n = 15), contralateral C7 (n = 16), ipsilateral C5–C6 (n = 5), and spinal accessory nerve (n = 2). Donor motor nerves chosen to restore finger extension included intercostals (n = 14), contralateral C7 (n = 12), spinal accessory nerve (n = 5), and ipsilateral plexus (n = 2). Overall, there was a significant improvement in mean muscle strength grading and joint range of motion for both finger flexion and extension. The graded muscle function and joint range of motion were greatest in patients who underwent spinal accessory neurotization; however, these differences were not found to be significantly different between the various donor motor nerves reviewed. More recent literature has challenged the use of contralateral C7 in brachial plexus reconstruction owing to poor reported outcomes and the potential for significant donor site morbidity.[19]

## DONOR MUSCLE

Understanding muscle physiology is important when performing the functional muscle transfer. Skeletal muscle contraction relies on the overlapping effects of myosin and actin filaments. These molecules are overlapped to some degree at a resting state and their interconnections allow them to slide across each other during muscle contraction. Skeletal muscle properties rely on restoration of this length-tension relationship; therefore, it is important to set the muscle resting tension appropriately to maximize muscle contraction forces. The muscle resting length maximizes the actin and myosin overlap and therefore the potential muscle contraction strength. Overtensioning or undertensioning of the muscle can therefore weaken the muscle contraction force. Terzis and Kostopoulos[18] described their technique of determining the resting tension of the muscles by placing a series of sutures spaced 1 cm apart along the entire muscle to be transferred. The muscle is then released from its origin and insertion site, leading to a notable contraction that can be challenging to restore. Using the technique of Terzis and Kostopoulos,[18] the muscle is simply stretched at its recipient site until the 1-cm suture intervals are reestablished.

There are a number of available donor muscle options for upper extremity functional reconstruction. When choosing a donor, the ideal muscle should be powerful and long enough to accomplish the recipient site function desired. It should be kept in mind that the maximum muscle force is determined by the muscle's cross-sectional area, whereas the muscle fiber length determines the overall range at which the muscle can generate a forced contracture.[20] Furthermore, the muscle chosen should have available tendon and fascia to support origin and insertion attachments. In situations in which these supporting structures are inadequate, Shridharani and colleagues[21] advocated the use of a gastrointestinal stapler across the muscle to provide additional strength and suture-holding capabilities. One must also consider the neurovascular anatomy of the transplanted muscle. Mathes and Nahai Types 1 (single dominant pedicle), 2 (single dominant pedicle and minor pedicles), and 5 (single dominant pedicle and segmental pedicles) muscles with a dominant vascular pedicle should be considered for free functional muscle transfer. The pedicle length should be adequate to allow microvascular anastomosis outside the zone of injury and ischemic soft tissue bed while also allowing an appropriate and match of caliber size. When considering the donor defect, the ideal donor site should not leave too great a functional loss, and the incision should be easily disguised. Last, the donor muscle should have a single motor nervous supply. There are a number of available muscles that meet many of these criteria and can be considered in free functional muscle transfers. These include the gracilis, latissimus dorsi, tensor fascia latae, rectus femoris, medial gastrocnemius, serratus anterior, and the pectoralis major/minor. The gracilis and latissimus dorsi also can be harvested as a myocutaneous flap with a reliable skin paddle to provide additional soft tissue coverage while also allowing primary donor site closure. The gracilis muscle is considered at most institutions to be the gold standard donor muscle. The gracilis functions to flex, medially rotate, and adduct the thigh, although its sacrifice does not result in any apparent functional deficit.

## SURGICAL TECHNIQUE FOR GRACILIS MUSCLE HARVEST

The patient is positioned supine or slightly lateral with the contralateral side elevated. The anticipated leg for harvest is placed in a frog lateral position. The incision is designed and a line is drawn from the pubic tubercle to the medial condyle. When a skin paddle is to be included, it is designed in the proximal one-third of the leg and just posterior to the line that is drawn so as to capture more reliable cutaneous perforators. With the leg placed in a hyperabducted position, the adductor longus tendon is easily palpated proximally in the medial thigh and will guide the proximal gracilis dissection. The incision is made along the entire length of the muscle as the proximal fascial origin and the distal tendon are harvested with the muscle. The sartorius muscle is identified crossing from the anterior thigh to the medial condyle, as the gracilis muscle is the posterior-most adductor of the thigh. The correct muscle is confirmed by noting that the origin of the gracilis is the pubic tubercle, whereas the origin of the sartorius is the anterior superior iliac spine. The medial thigh fascia is incised and left incorporated with the gracilis muscle allowing potentially improved muscle contraction and tendon gliding. The distal tendon is identified and further lengthened by its separation from the pes anserinus. Once the muscle and distal insertion have been confirmed, the dissection is carried proximally to identify the neurovascular pedicle. Leaving the muscle attached distal and proximal will aid in the proximal neurovascular pedicle dissection by providing tension on the muscle and allowing better confirmation of muscle stimulation once the obturator nerve is stimulated. The muscle is marked (as described by Terzis and colleagues) with a series of sutures or hemo-clips every 1 to 5 cm, which are later used as a guide for restoring muscle length/tension.[13,18] The vascular pedicle is typically identified 8 to 12 cm distal to the pubic tubercle. The anterior branch of the obturator nerve is identified on the medial surface of the muscle just proximal (superior) to the medial circumflex artery and vein (**Fig. 1**). The average nerve length that can be taken with the flap is approximately 7 cm. The artery and vein can be further dissected to their origin at the profunda femoris artery often requiring ligation of

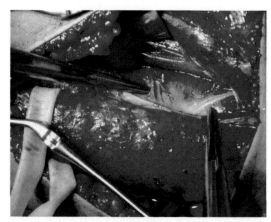

**Fig. 1.** The gracilis muscle is dissected with attention to the vascular pedicle and anterior branch of the obturator nerve, which can be seen on the medial surface of the muscle just proximal to the pedicle. (*Courtesy of Jeffrey Marcus, MD, Durham, NC.*)

muscular perforators to the adductor longus muscle. The artery is typically 6 cm in length and 1 to 2 mm in vessel diameter. The artery is accompanied by 2 venae comitantes each measuring 1 to 4 mm in diameter.

Before artery and vein ligation, the obturator nerve is stimulated. The gracilis muscle will typically contract 50% of the resting length or 12 to 15 cm in total contraction length. The obturator nerve to the gracilis muscle is typically supplied by 2 to 3 major fascicles. An intrafascicular dissection can be performed with one fascicle isolated and noted to control the anterior 20% to 50% of the muscle while the remaining fascicles are noted to control the posterior portion of the muscle. This split in muscle innervation can be used in scenarios to control thumb flexion and independent finger flexion.[22]

## SURGICAL TECHNIQUE FOR FREE FUNCTIONAL MUSCLE TRANSFER FOR ELBOW FLEXION

Selection of the donor motor nerve occurs in the preoperative timeframe. Ideally, a single motor nerve should be chosen to provide muscle reinnervation. The preferred motor nerve following trauma, oncologic resections, or ischemic muscle loss includes a motor branch of the musculocutaneous, motor branches from the ulnar nerve, the spinal accessory nerve, or the medial or lateral pectoral nerve. Alternatively, patients who are considered for free functional transfer to restore elbow flexion who have sustained severe brachial plexus injuries will have a paucity of donor motor nerves available. The intercostals have been used with the greatest experience and may contain between 1200 and 1300 myelinated axonal fibers, which is adequate to innervate a free functional muscle transfer. Kay and colleagues[23] reported an experience of 33 gracilis free muscle transfers and demonstrated improved muscle strength in patients treated with intercostal donor motor nerves when compared with ulnar motor nerves. In comparison, Hattori and colleagues[24] demonstrated improved muscle cross-sectional area and strength in muscles treated with the spinal accessory nerve when compared with intercostal nerves. Harvesting the intercostal nerves is not without potential complications. Kovachevich and colleagues[25] reviewed 153 brachial plexus reconstructions with intercostal motor nerves and demonstrated an overall complication rate of 15%, with pleural tears being the most common occurrence. These investigators also found that the rate of complications increased with increasing numbers of intercostals harvested.

The second to fourth intercostal nerves are commonly used, given their close proximity to the upper extremity and may have the opportunity to be coapted without the use of a nerve graft. The chest wall skin incision is planned in line with the third rib, which allows access to the adjacent superior and inferior ribs. The skin and subcutaneous tissue are first dissected, followed by the superficial muscular layer, which exposes the intercostal space. The nerve is then located in the muscular layers between the intercostalis intimi and internal intercostal muscles (**Fig. 2**). Each of the nerves is cut as close to the midline of the chest as possible and brought together at the lateral aspect of the chest wall. The nerves can be brought together with suture or the use of a nerve conduit.

An extensile upper arm incision is designed to include exposure of the lateral clavicle and acromion. It then extends toward the medial epicondyle and crosses the antecubital fossa into the forearm. Dissection typically starts in an area without previous injury or scar tissue. Adequate vessels for anastomosis should be identified before donor flap artery ligation. The thoracoacromial, lateral thoracic, and subscapular arteries are excellent size matched options, or alternatively, the brachial artery can be used with an end-to-side anastomosis. The skin is incised and elevated in the subcutaneous plane or a pocket is created to allow local soft tissue coverage over the functional free muscle transfer. The gracilis muscle can be harvested with a cutaneous paddle when additional soft tissue coverage is needed.

The lateral clavicle and acromion are prepared for the gracilis muscle origin. Nonabsorbable sutures can be placed in the periosteum, or the muscle can be directly attached to the bone with either suture anchors or bone tunnels. With the origin of the muscle secure, the muscle is then stretched out to its resting tension and length (restoring the previously placed 1-cm markers) and the vascular pedicle and nerve position are judged. The vascular anastomoses are then performed under microscope magnification. With the origin of the muscle secure and vascular perfusion restored, the distal biceps tendon is dissected and the gracilis muscle is pulled out to length. The approximate site of tendon repair is then marked with the elbow held in full extension. The elbow is then temporarily flexed and the tendon repair is performed with a Pulvertaft weave using nonabsorbable suture. Finally, the chosen motor nerve is coapted to the obturator nerve as close to the muscle as possible so as decrease reinnervation time.

Postoperatively, patients are placed in a splint for 3 weeks supporting the elbow in flexion so as to avoid excessive tension on the tendon repair. Patients are then involved in a gentle passive range of motion stretching program. Once the muscle becomes innervated, patients will begin cortical reeducation as they learn to flex the elbow with deep inspiration (in scenarios in which the intercostals are used). Over time, inspiratory efforts to drive the muscle action potential are no longer necessary. Chalidapong and colleagues[26] showed that trunk flexion and learned elbow flexion showed maximum amplitudes on electrodiagnostic evaluation when compared with forced inspiration or expiration.

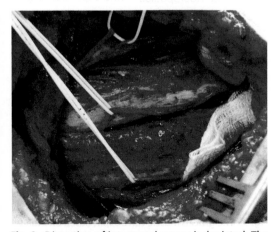

**Fig. 2.** Dissection of intercostal nerves is depicted. The motor branch of the intercostals can be located in the muscular layers between the intercostalis intimi and internal intercostal muscle.

## SURGICAL TECHNIQUE FOR FREE FUNCTIONAL MUSCLE TRANSFER FOR DIGIT FLEXION

Selection of the donor motor nerve is important to perform during in the preoperative time frame. It is preferred to select a single motor nerve (normally providing finger and wrist flexion) following trauma, oncologic resections, or Volkmann ischemic muscle contractures. Possibilities include the anterior interosseous branch of the median nerve, motor branches of the median nerve to the flexor digitorum superficialis, or branches of the ulnar nerve to the flexor digitorum profundus. In severe brachial plexopathies, Terzis and Kostopoulos[18] demonstrated good-to-excellent outcomes with the intercostals, contralateral C7 (which as noted previously has fallen out of favor), ipsilateral C5–C6, and spinal accessory nerves. Use of these alternative motor nerves does require an initial staged procedure that "banks" the nerve at the elbow, allowing it to mature through coapted nerve grafts.

An extensile forearm incision can be used to allow adequate exposure of the anticipated proximal muscle origin and the distal flexor tendons. The extensile approach is particularly important in patients with Volkmann contractures with anticipated extensive scar tissue. Dissection typically starts in an area without prior injury and an adequate vessel for anastomosis should be identified before donor flap artery ligation. In the region of the medial epicondyle, available arteries may consist of the ulnar recurrent, the anterior interosseous, or the larger caliber radial/ulnar proper arteries. The skin is elevated and a pocket is created to allow local soft tissue coverage over the functional free muscle transfer. Alternatively, the gracilis muscle can be harvested with a cutaneous paddle for added soft tissue coverage.

The distal flexor digitorum profundus tendons are then identified and prepared for tendon repair with the gracilis free functional muscle transfer. When a single muscle is used for digit flexion, each of the fingers should be tensioned to flex in concert so as to allow gripping of objects. The flexor digitorum profundus tendons are sutured together in a side-to-side technique with each adjacent ulnar digit in slightly more flexion. That is, the index finger should be balanced in the least flexion and the small digit is sutured with the greatest degree of flexion. The origin of the free muscle transfer is then inset either to the intermuscular septum or to the humerus by suture anchors or bone tunnels. The exact location of insetting depends on the overall length of the gracilis muscle that has been harvested. Terzis and

Kostopoulos[18] highlighted that most muscles are inset 12 to 15 cm proximal to the medial epicondyle. The vascular anastomoses are then performed under microscope magnification. With the origin of the muscle secure and vascular perfusion restored, the muscle is then stretched out to its resting tension and length (restoring the previously placed 1-cm markers) and a mark is placed on anticipated site of flexor tendon repair with the wrist and digits held in full extension. The wrist and digits are then brought into temporary flexion while the tendons are repaired using permanent suture and a Pulvertaft technique. The motor nerve is then prepared for coaptation. A nerve biopsy with carbonic anhydrase histochemistry can be performed to help delineate the differentiation of motor and sensory components.[18] The donor and recipient nerves should be cut to allow the coaptation to be as close to the muscle as possible to decrease the reinnervation time.

Balancing of the thumb can be challenging. When the thumb and digits are sutured to a single muscle transplant, the thumb should be sutured with some slack. The final outcome should demonstrate finger flexion that occurs before the initiation of thumb flexion to avoid a thumb-in-palm posture. Alternatively, Manktelow and Zuker,[22] in 1984, described a muscle splitting approach based on individual fascicular territories (Fig. 3). This could be used to provide thumb flexion that is independent of finger flexion.

Postoperatively, the patients are placed in a dorsal-based wrist and hand splint to avoid excessive tension on the tendon repair site. A continuous passive motion device can be used in the early postoperative time period or the patient can participate in therapy-based passive motion. Terzis and Kostopoulos[18] advocate the use of

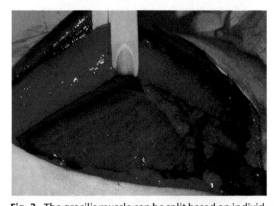

**Fig. 3.** The gracilis muscle can be split based on individual fascicular innervation. The vascular pedicle and obturator nerve are depicted superiorly. The muscle has been split based on its fascicular innervation. (*Courtesy of* Jeffrey Marcus, MD, Durham, NC.)

slow pulse muscle stimulation starting at 6 weeks for 5 to 6 hours per day until active motor function is demonstrated.

## REPORTED OUTCOMES

Variable reported outcomes of free functional muscle transfers are related to the indication in which they were performed. Free functional muscle transfers performed after Volkmann contractures and trauma are reported to outperform those following brachial plexus injuries. This discrepancy is related to the extent axonal input and muscle reinnervation provided by the available donor motor nerve. Becker and colleagues[27] examined the histology of free functional muscle transfers by biopsies performed during secondary procedures. These investigators found that patients with Muscle Grade 4 strength showed that the average muscle reinnervation was 46% in comparison with 31%, 24%, and 21% in muscles with Grades 3, 2, and 1 strength, respectively. These investigators concluded that the muscle force generated depended on the quality of the nerve regeneration. Kauhanen and colleagues[28] performed a similar study with biopsies of muscles performed 3 to 4 years postoperative. These investigators found that 64% of specimens demonstrated severe muscle atrophy of slow-type fibers. They also showed evidence of neuronal immunohistochemistry markers (PGP 9.5 and S-100) in muscles 3 to 4 years after the index procedure, suggesting a continued attempt at further reinnervation. Changes at the neuromuscular junction may also contribute to the lack of full muscle recovery. Hua and colleagues[29] in an animal study examined the neuromuscular junctions following gracilis free muscle transfers. Specimens with axonal loss demonstrated evidence of neuromuscular junction degeneration along with mitochondrial swelling and clumping. When reinnervation was established, specimens then showed regeneration of newly formed neuromuscular junctions in the same regions but with junctions that were smaller, had fewer structural details,[29] and fewer acetylcholine receptors.[30] These histologic changes correlate with the findings seen on MRI with transplanted muscles showing an increased proportion of fat and deceased muscle tissue in patients with clinically poor functional outcomes.[31]

Zuker and colleagues[12] reported on 7 patients with ischemic Volkmann contractures who underwent gracilis free muscle transfer. Patients had dramatic improvements in hand function following muscle transfer but with grip strengths of 25% of the contralateral uninjured side. Chuang[32] also reported on 47 free functional muscle transfers but

excluded patients with brachial plexus injuries. Most patients were either treated for Volkmann ischemic contractures or severe upper extremity crush/traction injuries and showed significant restorations in hand function.[32] In an earlier article, these same investigators found improved outcomes following free functional muscle transfers in patients with Volkmann ischemia who were treated with early (less than 3 weeks) exploration and muscle debridement in an attempt to remove the ischemic tissue and prevent severe fibrosis.[33]

Sterling Bunnell's classic phrase, "To someone who has nothing, a little is a lot" is no truer than in patients undergoing free functional muscle transfers following severe brachial plexus injuries.[34] Barrie and colleagues[35] reported on 29 free functional muscle transfers, with most neurotizations from intercostal nerves and showed Muscle Grade 4 or Muscle Grade 5 strength in 55%. Better outcomes occurred when a single muscle was used for a single function as opposed to 2 functions (elbow flexion and wrist extension). Terzis and Kostopoulos[13] reported on a larger, more heterogeneous patient population showing significantly improved postoperative strength following gracilis free muscle transfers neurotized with intercostals for elbow flexion but with a postoperative mean Muscle Grade between 2 and 3. These same investigators demonstrated similar findings in patients treated for finger flexion and extension with significantly improved postoperative Muscle Grades but at a mean of 3.2 (finger flexion) and 2.4 (finger extension) when the free functional muscle was neurotized with intercostals.[18]

## SUMMARY

Free functional muscle transfers should be considered in patients who have either failed or are not deemed to be candidates for local muscle/tendon transfers or neurotization procedures. Improved outcomes have been reported for trauma and Volkmann contracture etiologies secondary to improved muscle reinnervation potential. Free functional muscle transfers for complete brachial plexus injuries remain a powerful reconstructive tool to restore lost upper extremity function.

## REFERENCES

1. Gutowski KA, Orenstein HH. Restoration of elbow flexion after brachial plexus injury: the role of nerve and muscle transfers. Plast Reconstr Surg 2000; 106(6):1348–57 [quiz: 1358; discussion: 1359].
2. Terzis JK, Vekris MD, Soucacos PN. Outcomes of brachial plexus reconstruction in 204 patients with

devastating paralysis. Plast Reconstr Surg 1999; 104(5):1221–40.

3. Tamai S, Komatsu S, Sakamoto H, et al. Free muscle transplants in dogs, with microsurgical neurovascular anastomoses. Plast Reconstr Surg 1970;46(3): 219–25.

4. Terzis JK, Sweet RC, Dykes RW, et al. Recovery of function in free muscle transplants using microneurovascular anastomoses. J Hand Surg Am 1978;3(1): 37–59.

5. Stevanovic MV, Seaber AV, Urbaniak JR. Canine experimental free muscle transplantation. Microsurgery 1986;7(3):105–13.

6. Manktelow RT, McKee NH. Free muscle transplantation to provide active finger flexion. J Hand Surg Am 1978;3(5):416–26.

7. Ikuta Y, Yoshioka K, Tsuge K. Free muscle graft as applied to brachial plexus injury—case report and experimental study. Ann Acad Med Singapore 1979;8(4):454–8.

8. Stevanovic M, Sharpe F. Functional free muscle transfer for upper extremity reconstruction. Plast Reconstr Surg 2014;134(2):257e–74e.

9. Doi K, Kuwata N, Kawakami F, et al. Limb-sparing surgery with reinnervated free-muscle transfer following radical excision of soft-tissue sarcoma in the extremity. Plast Reconstr Surg 1999;104(6): 1679–87.

10. Selber JC, Treadway C, Lopez A, et al. The use of free flap for limb salvage in children with tumors of the extremities. J Pediatr Surg 2011;46(4):736–44.

11. Serletti JM, Schingo VA Jr, Deuber MA, et al. Free tissue transfer in pediatric patients. Ann Plast Surg 1996;36(6):561–8.

12. Zuker RM, Egerszegi EP, Manktelow RT, et al. Volkmann's ischemic contracture in children: the results of free vascularized muscle transplantation. Microsurgery 1991;12(5):341–5.

13. Terzis JK, Kostopoulos VK. Free muscle transfer in posttraumatic plexopathies part II: the elbow. Hand (N Y) 2010;5(2):160–70.

14. Hattori Y, Doi K, Ikeda K, et al. Restoration of prehension using double free muscle technique after complete avulsion of brachial plexus in children: a report of three cases. J Hand Surg Am 2005;30(4): 812–9.

15. Doi K, Sakai K, Kuwata N, et al. Reconstruction of finger and elbow function after complete avulsion of the brachial plexus. J Hand Surg Am 1991; 16(5):796–803.

16. Doi K, Muramatsu K, Hattori Y, et al. Restoration of prehension with the double free muscle technique following complete avulsion of the brachial plexus. Indications and long-term results. J Bone Joint Surg Am 2000;82(5):652–66.

17. Doi K, Kuwata N, Muramatsu K, et al. Double muscle transfer for upper extremity reconstruction following complete avulsion of the brachial plexus. Hand Clin 1999;15(4):757–67.

18. Terzis JK, Kostopoulos VK. Free muscle transfer in posttraumatic plexopathies: part III. The hand. Plast Reconstr Surg 2009;124(4):1225–36.

19. Sammer DM, Kircher MF, Bishop AT, et al. Hemi-contralateral C7 transfer in traumatic brachial plexus injuries: outcomes and complications. J Bone Joint Surg Am 2012;94(2):131–7.

20. Lieber RL. Skeletal muscle architecture: implications for muscle function and surgical tendon transfer. J Hand Ther 1993;6(2):105–13.

21. Shridharani SM, Stapleton SM, Redett RJ, et al. Use of gastrointestinal anastomosis stapler for harvest of gracilis muscle and securing it in the face for facial reanimation: a novel technique. Eplasty 2010;10:e29.

22. Manktelow RT, Zuker RM. Muscle transplantation by fascicular territory. Plast Reconstr Surg 1984;73(5): 751–7.

23. Kay S, Pinder R, Wiper J, et al. Microvascular free functioning gracilis transfer with nerve transfer to establish elbow flexion. J Plast Reconstr Aesthet Surg 2010;63(7):1142–9.

24. Hattori Y, Doi K, Ikedu K, et al. Ultrasonographic evaluation of functioning free muscle transfer: comparison between spinal accessory and intercostal nerve reinnervation. J Reconstr Microsurg 2006; 22(6):423–7.

25. Kovachevich R, Kircher MF, Wood CM, et al. Complications of intercostal nerve transfer for brachial plexus reconstruction. J Hand Surg Am 2010; 35(12):1995–2000.

26. Chalidapong P, Sananpanich K, Klaphajone J. Electromyographic comparison of various exercises to improve elbow flexion following intercostal nerve transfer. J Bone Joint Surg Br 2006;88(5):620–2.

27. Becker MH, Wermter TB, Brenner B, et al. Comparison of clinical performance, histology and single-fiber contractility in free neurovascular muscle flaps. J Reconstr Microsurg 2000;16(7):525–34.

28. Kauhanen MS, Lorenzetti F, Leivo IV, et al. Long-term morphometric and immunohistochemical findings in human free microvascular muscle flaps. Microsurgery 2004;24(1):30–8.

29. Hua J, Kumar VP, Tay SS, et al. Microscopic changes at the neuromuscular junction in free muscle transfer. Clin Orthop Relat Res 2003;(411): 325–33.

30. Hua J, Samuel TS, Kumar VP. Qualitative and quantitative changes in acetylcholine receptor distribution at the neuromuscular junction following free muscle transfer. Muscle Nerve 2002;25(3):427–32.

31. Yla-Kotola TM, Kauhanen MS, Koskinen SK, et al. Magnetic resonance imaging of microneurovascular free muscle flaps in facial reanimation. Br J Plast Surg 2005;58(1):22–7.

32. Chuang DC. Functioning free-muscle transplantation for the upper extremity. Hand Clin 1997;13(2):279–89.

33. Chuang DC, Carver N, Wei FC. A new strategy to prevent the sequelae of severe Volkmann's ischemia. Plast Reconstr Surg 1996;98(6):1023–31 [discussion: 1032–3].

34. Shin AY. 2004-2005 Sterling Bunnell Traveling Fellowship report. J Hand Surg Am 2006;31(7):1226–37.

35. Barrie KA, Steinmann SP, Shin AY, et al. Gracilis free muscle transfer for restoration of function after complete brachial plexus avulsion. Neurosurg Focus 2004;16(5):E8.

# Tendon Transfers in the Rheumatoid Hand for Reconstruction

Michael Brody O'Sullivan, MD, Hardeep Singh, MD,
Jennifer Moriatis Wolf, MD*

## KEYWORDS

- Rheumatoid arthritis • Tendon rupture • Tendon transfer • Hand

## KEY POINTS

- Patients with rheumatoid arthritis–induced tendon rupture frequently present in a delayed fashion. Tendinous invasion by inflammatory tissue is common. As such, primary tendon repair is not often possible.
- Tendon transfers are the first-line treatment of patients with rheumatoid arthritis–induced tendon ruptures. However, if a transfer is not possible, tendon grafting may serve a role.
- At the time of surgery, the underlying cause of the rupture should be addressed to prevent future additional tendon ruptures.
- Patients presenting with multiple ruptures typically experience worse outcomes and may require multiple different surgical procedures to restore function.

## INTRODUCTION

Rheumatoid arthritis is an autoimmune disease that affects approximately 2% of people more than 60 years of age in the United States.[1] The disease is caused by the so-called rheumatoid factor, a circulating immunoglobulin M molecule with affinity for self-immunoglobulin G molecules. Depositions of rheumatoid factor stimulate macrophage activity, resulting in a cascade of inflammation. Increased levels of proinflammatory cytokines and cells lead to local destruction of the synovial contents. Pannus formation, or synovial hyperplasia, results from this chronic inflammatory response. Over time, chronic erosive changes of the joints lead to soft tissue and bony deformity with formation of bony prominences or spicules, which may cause tendon attrition and later rupture. In addition, synovitis can infiltrate the substance of the tendons, which weakens them. With compromised tendon integrity caused by this chronic inflammation as well as local tendon irritation secondary to bony prominences, rheumatoid patients frequently develop tendon ruptures.

In the past 15 years there have been significant advances in the medical treatment of rheumatoid arthritis. The increased use of disease-modifying antirheumatic drugs (DMARDs) and the introduction of biologic DMARDs have resulted in a greater proportion of patients experiencing remission or lower disease activity status.[2,3] The increasing use of these agents has resulted in lower rates of progression of radiographic disease in a prospective observational study following patients for 10 years.[2]

At present, it is not known whether the improvements in medical management of this disease can influence the rates of tendon rupture. In an observational series of patients who experienced a

Disclosures: The authors have no significant financial information to disclose.
Department of Orthopaedic Surgery, University of Connecticut Health Center, 263 Farmington Avenue, Farmington, CT 06030, USA
* Corresponding author. University of Connecticut, 263 Farmington Avenue, Farmington, CT 06030.
E-mail address: jmwhand@gmail.com

Hand Clin 32 (2016) 407–416
http://dx.doi.org/10.1016/j.hcl.2016.03.014

rheumatoid-induced tendon rupture from 2005 to 2010, Gong and colleagues[4] noted no difference in the number of tendons ruptured, radiographic rheumatoid arthritis severity, and disease duration between 24 patients who were treated for their disease medically and 14 patients who were not. Tendon rupture is a late complication of the disease often presenting a decade or later after diagnosis.[5] Given that medical treatment has been shown to reduce disease activity and that the rates of radiographic rheumatoid arthritis severity were similar between groups in this study, the initiation of medical treatment of the patients in this series likely occurred too late in the disease process to affect the incidence of tendon rupture. With the advances in the medical management of these patients, the incidence of tendon rupture may significantly decrease in the future.

## DIAGNOSIS

Tendon ruptures present when a patient notes a sudden inability to flex or extend a finger or thumb. In a rheumatoid population, these ruptures are often painless and occur during routine use. These ruptures frequently go unnoticed for some time because of the patients' baseline functional limitations, causing a delayed presentation for medical evaluation.[5–8]

Diagnosis of a tendon rupture in a rheumatoid population requires a thorough history and physical examination. Preexisting deformity and concomitant disorders, including limitations in joint range of motion, can make the diagnosis a challenge. When a patient presents with the inability to flex or extend a digit, alternative diagnoses must first be excluded based on physical examination. Such diagnoses include:

- Tenosynovitis
- Sagittal band rupture
- Metacarpophalangeal (MCP) joint dislocation
- Posterior interosseous nerve (PIN) palsy

Sagittal band rupture is typically a radial-sided tear manifested by ulnar dislocation of the extensor tendon. Patients with either a sagittal band rupture or an extensor tendon rupture lose the ability to actively extend the digit. However, patients with a sagittal band rupture maintain the ability to hold their digits extended against gravity after passive extension, and those with extensor rupture cannot. Patients presenting with MCP joint dislocation have negligible passive range of motion of the joint, in contrast with patients with a tendon rupture. These dislocations can also be identified on standard radiographic images. In addition, patients with rheumatoid arthritis may also present with elbow synovitis causing a PIN palsy.[9] This diagnosis should be suspected, as opposed to multiple extensor tendon ruptures, when passive tenodesis, or passive finger extension with passive wrist flexion, shows symmetric extension and flexion.[7,9]

## TENDON GRAFTING VERSUS TENDON TRANSFER

In certain scenarios, tendon grafting may be appropriate for reconstruction following an extensor or flexor tendon rupture. With chronic ruptures, the proximal motor unit becomes contracted and develops adhesions rendering it nonfunctional. However, the literature regarding the optimal timing for tendon grafting in a rheumatoid population is not well defined. Magnell and colleagues[10] reported on a series of 21 patients who underwent tendon grafting for extensor pollicis longus (EPL) reconstruction. They stated that acceptable results were obtained up to 21 weeks postrupture. However, this series included only 2 patients with rheumatoid arthritis who underwent surgical intervention at 1 and 4 weeks postrupture. Chung and colleagues[5] showed good results in a series of 28 rheumatoid patients treated with tendon grafting at an average of 18 weeks postrupture. In contrast, Nakamura and Katsuki[11] noted an unacceptable loss of finger flexion with an average postoperative fingertip-to-palm distance of 1.6 cm when performing tendon grafting on 14 patients with rheumatoid arthritis–induced extensor tendon ruptures at an average of 12 weeks. These investigators noted that intraoperative tendon excursion of the proximal motor unit was greater than 2 cm in all cases and their grafts were sewn with greater tension than those of previous investigators, suggesting that graft overtensioning rather than muscle contracture may have caused the suboptimal clinical outcomes. Taken together, these findings suggest that tendon grafting may be possible up to 20 weeks postrupture in rheumatoid patients.

Some investigators have suggested that tendon grafts are prone to adhesion formation in rheumatoid tissue and should be avoided.[7,8,12] However, this recommendation consists of expert opinion and primary literature is lacking. Meanwhile, others have shown good functional results and improved biomechanical properties using tendon grafting for the repair of extensor tendon ruptures in this patient population.[13,14]

Comparative studies between tendon grafting and tendon transfer for the repair of extensor tendon ruptures in rheumatoid patients are lacking in the literature. One retrospective review comparing 11 cases of tendon transfer with 28 cases of tendon grafting noted no significant difference in clinical results.[5] Further study is required to better define the role of tendon grafting in the treatment of patients with rheumatoid arthritis.

In the absence of definitive literature, the authors think that tendon transfer should serve as the first-line treatment of tendon ruptures in rheumatoid patients. Patients with rheumatoid arthritis are known to have impaired wound healing capability.[15] Assuming that a redundant tendon with low donor site morbidity is available for transfer, tendon transfer is preferred to tendon grafting because it avoids concerns over the competency of the proximal muscular unit and requires the patient to heal only 1 site of repair. However, if a tendon is not available for transfer, as can be the case in the setting of multiple ruptures, tendon grafting may provide the best option for functional recovery. Choices for tendon donors include:

- Palmaris longus
- Strips of extensor carpi radialis brevis or extensor carpi radialis longus (ECRL)
- Plantaris
- Extensor tendon to the fourth toe[8,10,13,14]

## EXTENSOR TENDON RUPTURES
### Extensor Pollicis Longus Ruptures

The EPL tendon is frequently ruptured in patients with rheumatoid arthritis. These ruptures typically occur at the Lister tubercle, caused by attritional damage. The EPL provides extension at both the interphalangeal (IP) and MCP joints of the thumb. However, the functional limitation following EPL rupture is variable. With a rupture in the EPL, patients typically retain some extension at the MCP joint through the action of the extensor pollicis brevis (EPB) and the IP joint through the thumb intrinsics. Nevertheless, extension at the MCP joint is often weak and functionally limiting.[7,8]

Primary repair with healthy edges of the EPL tendon is typically not possible because of significant gapping, because rheumatoid patients tend to present for evaluation in a delayed fashion and because the disease alters the tendon composition.[6] Isolated EPL ruptures are commonly treated with an extensor indicis proprius (EIP) tendon transfer (**Fig. 1**). The EIP is suitable for tendon transfer because:

- It provides a redundant function, extending the index finger
- It has the length necessary to reach the thumb or the small finger
- It acts independently[6]

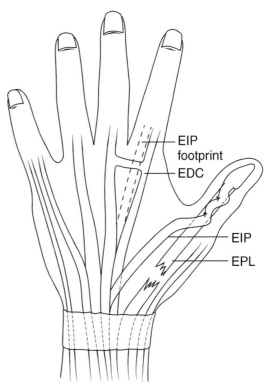

**Fig. 1.** Transfer of the EIP tendon to the ruptured EPL for restoration of extensor function in the setting of a ruptured EPL. EDC, extensor digitorum communis.

- In addition, the EPL and the EIP have similar tendon excursion (5.8 cm vs 5.4 cm), direction of pull, muscle strength (0.3 kg*m vs 0.5 kg*m), and size.[16]

Before any EIP transfer, the integrity of the index finger extensor digitorum communis (EDC) tendon must be assessed. If the index finger EDC tendon is incompetent, an EIP transfer should not be attempted. In addition, evaluation of the thumb for preexisting boutonniere or swan-neck deformity is critical, because tendon transfer in this scenario may not improve function. If the patient has chronic boutonniere or swan-neck deformity, fusion of the MCP or IP joints or both may be considered if splinting proves insufficient.

When the EIP tendon is harvested immediately proximal to the extensor hood, this tendon can be transferred without any resultant functional limitation in the index finger.[17,18] The EIP runs on the ulnar aspect of the index finger at the level of the MCP joint. Proximally, this muscle passes through the fourth dorsal compartment at the level of the wrist and has the most distal muscle belly, which confirms identification.[7] After harvesting, the musculotendinous unit is withdrawn to the level of the wrist, passed subcutaneously, and secured to the EPL tendon stump via a Pulvertaft weave.[19,20] EIP-to-EPL transfer has shown excellent clinical outcomes, recreating 86% of the pinch strength and 92% of the grip strength of the contralateral uninvolved extremity in patients with rheumatoid arthritis.[21]

In the setting of multiple tendon ruptures, the EIP may be needed for transfer to the ulnar digits or may not be available for transfer, having previously ruptured or providing sole index finger extension. Magnell and colleagues[10] showed good results with tendon grafting for EPL repair with a competent proximal musculotendinous unit within 21 weeks of rupture. If the proximal unit shows less than 2 cm of tendon excursion intraoperatively or the rupture is more chronic in nature, irreversible contracture and adhesion formation should be assumed and grafting should be avoided.[10,11] However, this study included only 2 patients with rheumatoid arthritis and it may not be possible to generalize the results to the rheumatoid population.[10] Transfer of the abductor pollicis longus (APL) has been described for EPL ruptures in rheumatoid patients. Although this tendon has significantly less excursion (2.8 cm vs 5.4 cm) than the EIP,[16] Backhouse[22] reported similar results with transfer of the APL, assuming the distal tendon stump has sufficient length for repair. Partial transfer of the ECRL has also been described. Despite the reduced tendon excursion of the ECRL compared with the EPL (3.7 cm vs 5.8 cm), Chetta and colleagues[16] showed that treatment of an EPL rupture with a partial turn-down transfer of the ECRL in a case study resulted in identical grip strength and slightly reduced pinch strength compared with the contralateral extremity. In addition, Harrison and colleagues[23] advocated an EPB-to-EPL transfer to preserve abduction of the thumb during extension for pinch strength. The investigators stated that satisfactory results were obtained with this transfer. However, this procedure does not address the weakness in extension at the MCP joint after EPL rupture.

## PROCEDURE: EXTENSOR INDICIS PROPRIUS TO EXTENSOR POLLICIS LONGUS TENDON TRANSFER
### Preoperative Planning and Patient Positioning

Before any surgical intervention, a thorough history and physical should be obtained. Radiographs of the cervical spine should be considered to rule out instability before surgery. The surgeon should coordinate with the patient's rheumatologist to withhold certain anti–tumor necrosis factor DMARDs, because these have been postulated to increase risk for surgical site infection.[24] Before undertaking a tendon transfer, the surgeon should develop a plan with consideration of which tendons are involved, which tendons are available for transfer, the duration of tendon incompetence, and the concomitant disorder.[20]

The patient is positioned supine with the hand on a radiolucent hand table. Anesthesia options include local anesthesia combined with monitored anesthesia care to allow for assessment of tenodesis and tendon gliding intraoperatively, regional block, or general anesthesia. A tourniquet should be applied to ensure a bloodless surgical field. If considering tendon grafting, the contralateral extremity can be draped for access.[20]

- Step 1: through a 1-cm to 2-cm longitudinal incision on the dorsal aspect of the index finger MCP, identify the EIP tendon on the ulnar aspect as it inserts into the extensor hood.
- Step 2: create a 3-cm to 4-cm longitudinal incision over the dorsal aspect of the distal radius just ulnar to the Lister tubercle.
- Step 3: dissect through the extensor retinaculum and into the fourth dorsal compartment.
- Step 4: identify and isolate the EIP tendon at the dorsal wrist. The tendon has the most distal muscle belly and is located deep to the EDC tendons. Confirm the identification by placing tension on the distal and proximal aspects of the tendon.
- Step 5: transect the EIP tendon immediately proximal to its insertion into the extensor hood and withdraw the tendon from the dorsal wrist incision. If maximal length is needed, the graft can be harvested with a portion of the extensor hood and the sagittal band advanced to close the gap.
- Step 6: create a 4-cm incision over the dorsal aspect of the thumb proximal to the MCP joint in line with the EPL tendon.
- Step 7: suture the distal end of the EIP tendon to a pediatric feeding tube. Pass the feeding tube subcutaneously from the dorsal wrist through the thumb incision. With the EIP tendon exposed in the dorsal thumb incision, cut the sutures to remove the feeding tube.
- Step 8: secure the EIP tendon to the distal aspect of the ruptured EPL tendon using a Pulvertaft weave, using nonabsorbable or slowly absorbing, undyed 2-0 suture. Adjust tension so that full extension is obtained with wrist flexion.
- Step 9: irrigate and close the wounds. Apply a sterile dressing and a thumb spica splint with the IP joint slightly hyperextended.[20]

## Postoperative Management

Most investigators recommend a period of immobilization followed by a gradual return to both passive and active motion following tendon transfer.[5,8,20] Typical postoperative recommendations include splinting the wrist in 40° of extension with the MCP joint held in slight flexion to avoid overtensioning the repair. The MCP joints should be held in flexion to avoid collateral ligament contracture.[8,20] IP joints can be kept free to allow for gentle range of motion immediately after surgery.[8,11,25] Typically, after a period of 3 to 4 weeks, a passive motion protocol is initiated, which is advanced to active motion and eventually slight resistance exercises by 6 weeks.[5,8,11,20] Dynamic extension splinting is another option applied at 3 weeks, used to slowly increase thumb flexion while protecting the transfer for 3 to 4 weeks.

## Isolated Tendon Ruptures

Rupture of the long extensor tendons to the fingers is a common sequela of rheumatoid arthritis. Vaughan-Jackson[26] first described the condition in 1948. Tendons can rupture because of invasion by inflammatory tissue or because of attrition.[6] With long-standing rheumatoid arthritis, the distal radial ulnar joint is affected by synovitis and joint destruction, ultimately destabilizing the joint. Over time, the distal ulna subluxates dorsally, abutting the overlying extensor tendons. As the extensor tendons glide across the inflamed dorsal radiocarpal synovium and eroded distal ulna, attrition of the extensors and ultimate ruptures can occur at this level. Because of its position in the fourth and fifth dorsal compartments, the extensor tendons to the small finger (EDC and extensor digiti quinti [EDQ]) are most commonly involved. Typically, ruptures begin in the ulnar digits and progress radially over time.[20,27]

As with any attempted tendon transfer, the underlying cause must be corrected at the time of surgery to prevent future ruptures. There are no large observational cohort studies to prove that operative intervention can prevent future tendon ruptures. However, there are case series in the literature that suggest that addressing the underlying cause of the rupture may reduce the rates of subsequent tendon rupture. Gong and colleagues[4] showed that 29 out of 38 (76%) patients had multiple tendon ruptures with an average time between subsequent ruptures of 2.9 months in their observational study of nonsurgically managed patients. In contrast, Millender and colleagues[12] showed that dorsal tenosynovectomy with or without a Darrach procedure in 93 patients

with rheumatoid arthritis yielded only 2 tendon ruptures at an average follow-up of 3 years. The investigators noted that 41 hands had tendon ruptures that were addressed at the time of surgery but did not specify whether the 2 patients with subsequent ruptures at follow-up were in this group. Taken together, these data suggest that surgical intervention designed to correct the underlying cause of tendon rupture may prevent or at least delay future ruptures. In the setting of an extensor tendon rupture, the preexisting rheumatoid synovitis and exposed ulnar head and bony spicules should be addressed surgically before performing a tendon transfer. This surgery may involve ulnar debridement or a formal Darrach procedure. In addition, the dorsal retinacular ligament can be sutured below the extensor tendons to provide a suitable tendon bed for a durable repair.[6,7]

The extensor tendons to the small finger are most commonly ruptured in patients with rheumatoid arthritis. An isolated EDQ rupture may not result in significant functional limitation, but nevertheless should be addressed surgically to prevent additional tendon ruptures.[12] Rupture of the EDQ results in a slight lag at the MCP joint, which is accentuated with MCP joint flexion of the index, middle, and ring fingers. Often, end-to-end repair is not possible with the remaining diseased tendon. As such, an end-to-side repair of the distal stump of the EDQ to the intact ring finger EDC tendon is recommended.[8,20]

With combined rupture of the EDQ and the small finger EDC tendon, patients are not able to extend the small finger at the MCP joint. In this scenario, an end-to-side repair of the distal stump of the small finger EDC/EDQ to the ring finger EDC tendon or an EIP to small finger EDC/EDQ transfer can be attempted. An EIP to small finger EDC/EDQ tendon transfer should be considered if rupture occurs distal to the midmetacarpal level, because an end-to-side repair in this scenario can result in forced abduction of the small finger.[20]

Although less common, isolated ruptures of the middle finger EDC and ring finger EDC tendons can occur. These ruptures are easily treated with end-to-side transfers to the EIP or middle finger EDC respectively. End-to-side transfers should occur in the radial direction such that ulnar deviation of the finger is not accentuated.

## PROCEDURE: END-TO-SIDE TENDON TRANSFER

- Step 1: create a 3-cm to 4-cm longitudinal incision centered between the metacarpal of the affected digit and the adjacent uninvolved digit.

- Step 2: locate the distal stump of the ruptured tendon and debride any inflamed tissue.
- Step 3: suture the distal tendon stump to the adjacent EDC tendon with nonabsorbable suture. Adjust tensioning such that full extension is achieved with wrist flexion, and digits are symmetrically aligned.
- Step 4: irrigate and close the surgical wound. Splint the involved 2 digits with the MCP joints held in extension and the IP joints free.

### Multiple Tendon Ruptures

Frequently, multiple tendons rupture in rheumatoid patients. Gong and colleagues[4] noted that 29 of 38 patients (76%) had ruptures in 2 or more digits in their series. The average time interval between first and subsequent ruptures was 2.9 months. Increased number of tendon ruptures and increased duration of rupture portend a worse prognosis.[28] When the ring and small tendons are incompetent, the ring finger can be repaired to the middle finger EDC tendon and the EIP tendon can be transferred to the small finger distal tendon stump (**Fig. 2**). Although an end-to-side repair of the small and ring finger EDC to the middle finger EDC tendon can be attempted, often the distal stump of the small finger EDC tendon is too short to bridge this gap. As such, performing an end-to-side transfer of the small finger to the middle finger may result in unacceptable abduction of the small finger.[6,7] Alternatively, an EIP to small finger and ring finger EDC can also be attempted (**Fig. 3**). **Table 1** shows the preferred treatment method for multiple different tendon rupture scenarios.

When the small, ring, and middle fingers are incompetent, the middle finger can be repaired to the index finger EDC in an end-to-side fashion and the EIP tendon can be transferred to power the ring finger and small finger tendon stumps. Suzuki and colleagues[25] performed a retrospective review of 48 patients presenting with triple tendon ruptures of the ulnar digits. Four techniques were evaluated, including a palmaris longus graft to the 3 extensor stumps, an EIP transfer to the 3 extensor tendon stumps, an end-to-side transfer of all 3 tendon stumps to the EIP or EDC in the index finger, and a combination of an end-to-side transfer of the middle finger EDC tendon to the index finger EDC with an EIP tendon transfer to the ring and small fingers. Clinical outcomes and MCP joint range of motion were best in the patients who underwent an end-to-side repair combined with an EIP tendon transfer.

When tendons to all 4 digits are incompetent, a flexor digitorum superficialis (FDS) transfer can be considered. Originally described by Boyes[29] and

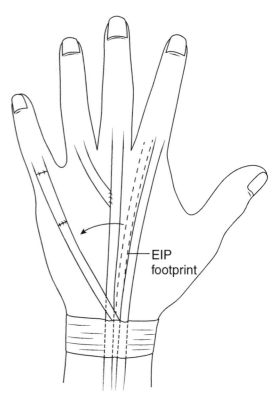

**Fig. 2.** Transfer of the EIP to the common extensor stump of the small finger with simultaneous end-to-side transfer of the ring finger tendon stump to the middle finger EDC tendon to restore extensor function in the setting of an EDQ, small finger EDC, and ring finger EDC tendon rupture.

subsequently modified by Nalebuff[6] and Nalebuff and Patel,[30] a dual FDS transfer can restore function (**Fig. 4**). The FDS tendons are ideal to transfer in this scenario because they serve a redundant function, show independent muscle contraction, have good length, and show good strength. Although these tendons provide an antagonistic function, patients can learn to use them following transfer.[6] The FDS tendon from the middle and ring fingers can be harvested immediately proximal to the tendon bifurcation, provided the patient has intact flexor digitorum profundus (FDP) tendons to each digit. The tendons are then accessed through a volar Henry approach, passing the tendons deep to the contents of the carpal tunnel and radial artery. In addition, the tendons are transferred dorsally across the radius, weaving the FDS of the middle finger to the EDC tendon stump of the index and middle finger and the FDS of the ring finger to the EDC tendon stump of the ring and small fingers.[20] Care must be taken not to overtension the transfer, which can result in impaired flexion.[6] With the wrist held in slight flexion, the fingers should obtain extension at the MCP joint.[20]

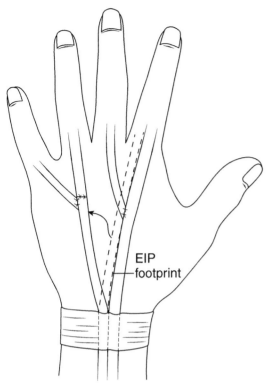

**Fig. 3.** Transfer of the EIP tendon to the small and ring finger extensor stumps for restoration of function following an EDQ, small finger EDC, and ring finger EDC tendon rupture.

## PROCEDURE: MIDDLE AND RING FLEXOR DIGITORUM SUPERFICIALIS TO INDEX THROUGH SMALL EXTENSOR DIGITORUM COMMUNIS TENDON TRANSFER

- Step 1: through a volar Henry approach, identify and isolate the FDS tendons to the middle and ring fingers. Placing tension on the intact tendons can aid in identification.
- Step 2: through 2 separate 1-cm oblique incisions over the volar aspect of the middle and ring fingers, dissect into the flexor tendon sheath.
- Step 3: identify the middle and ring finger FDS tendons and transect these tendons just proximal to their bifurcation through a window at the A3 pulley. This approach preserves the A1 pulley and may help to decrease ulnar drift.
- Step 4: withdraw the tendons through the volar wrist incision.
- Step 5: suture a pediatric feeding tube to the distal aspects of the middle and ring finger FDS tendons. Alternately, a tendon passer can be used from dorsal to volar.
- Step 6: create two 4-cm dorsal longitudinal incisions in the intermetacarpal space between the index and middle fingers and between the ring and small fingers.
- Step 7: using the feeding tubes, pass the tendons to the dorsal aspect of the radius keeping them deep to the FDP tendons, flexor pollicis longus (FPL) tendon, median nerve, and radial artery. Pass the middle finger FDS tendon

**Table 1**
**Surgical Options for Treatment of Tendon Ruptures in Patients with Rheumatoid Arthritis**

| Rupture | Treatment |
| --- | --- |
| EPL | First line: EIP tendon transfer<br>Second line (EIP unavailable for transfer): tendon grafting/APL transfer/partial ECRL transfer |
| EDQ | EDQ to SF EDC |
| EDQ + SF EDC | EDQ + SF EDC to RF EDC tendon transfer, or EIP tendon transfer |
| RF or MF EDC | EDC to adjacent radial EDC |
| EDQ + SF EDC + RF EDC | EIP to SF + RF EDC, or EIP to SF with RF EDC to MF EDC |
| RF and MF EDC | EIP tendon transfer |
| EDQ + SF EDC + RF EDC + MF EDC | EIP to SF + RF EDC with MF EDC to IF EDC |
| EDQ + SF EDC + RF EDC + MF EDC + IF EDC + EIP | MF FDS to IF and MF EDC with RF FDS to RF and SF EDC |
| FPL | FDS tendon transfer or tendon grafting or IP fusion |
| FDP | FDS tendon transfer or tendon grafting |

*Abbreviations:* FDP, flexor digitorum profundus; FDS, flexor digitorum superficialis; IF, index finger; MF, middle finger; RF, ring finger; SF, small finger.

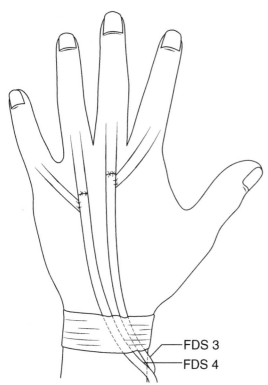

FDS 3

FDS 4

**Fig. 4.** Transfer of the middle and ring finger FDS tendons to restore extensor function following EDQ, small finger EDC, ring finger EDC, middle finger EDC, index finger EDC, and EIP tendon ruptures.

feeding tube through the incision between the index and middle fingers and the ring finger FDS tendon feeding tube through the incision between the ring and small fingers.

- Step 8: suture the tendon stumps of the index and middle fingers and the stumps of the ring and small fingers in a side-to-side or an end-to-side fashion.
- Step 9: suture the middle finger FDS tendon to the tendon stump of the index and middle fingers.
- Step 10: transfer the ring finger FDS tendon to the tendon stump of the ring and small fingers.
- Step 11: adjust tensioning such that the fingers obtain extension at the MCP joints with slight wrist flexion.
- Step 12: secure tendon transfer with a Pulver-taft weave.
- Step 13: irrigate and close wounds. Splint fingers with the MCP joints in extension and IP joints free.[6,20,30]

Literature comparing different postoperative motion protocols in patients with rheumatoid arthritis undergoing tendon transfer is minimal. Suzuki and colleagues[25] used immediate active motion in patients

who underwent an end-to-side tendon transfer in patients with multiple extensor tendon ruptures. The investigators taped the digit with the transferred tendon to an adjacent digit in a slightly extended position, similar to the extensor yoke splint proposed by Howell and colleagues[31] after tendon repair, and noted no complications with this protocol.

## FLEXOR TENDONS

Flexor tenosynovitis is a common finding in patients with rheumatoid arthritis and can be associated with joint involvement. Depending on the severity, rheumatoid flexor tenosynovitis can result in adhesion formation between the flexor mechanism and underlying bone and ligaments, leading to shortening and contracture formation, producing varying degrees of limitations in active and passive flexion.[32] However, flexor tendon ruptures are much less common than extensor tendon ruptures.[33,34] They are frequently associated with compression neuropathies because these have a high incidence in patients with rheumatoid arthritis.[34,35] The main causes of flexor tendon injuries in patients with rheumatoid arthritis are invasion of the tendons by an inflammatory synovial mass and attritional damage caused by bony spurs.[36] The proliferative synovitis leads to nodule formation changing the ultrastructure of the tendon, ultimately causing spontaneous rupture.[8] The attritional damage from a bony spur along with carpal instability in advanced rheumatoid wrist destruction leads to tendon rupture.[34,36] The common sites of tendon involvement are the volar aspect of the wrist and flexor tendons in the digital canal. Flexor tendon rupture presents with acute loss of flexion in 1 or more digits; however, diagnoses can be challenging in patients presenting with joint stiffness or instability.[32,33] Patients may initially present with trigger fingers, which has often been reported to be the earliest sign of the disease.[8] Ertel and colleagues[33] investigated 115 flexor tendon ruptures in 43 hands with rheumatoid arthritis, 1 hand with psoriatic arthritis, and 1 hand with lupus erythematosus. Most of the ruptures in this series were associated with damage from bony spurs, whereas the remainder were caused by synovitis. Ruptures occurred more frequently at the level of the wrist versus the digital canal. In this series, attritional ruptures tended to have improved motion versus those caused by invasion from tenosynovitis, isolated ruptures tended to have better functional results, and ruptures within the fibro-osseous canal had a poor prognosis. The investigators recommended prevention of tendon ruptures by early tenosynovectomy and removal of bone spurs.[33]

Tenosynovitis can present with difficulty in obtaining full finger flexion or triggering of the affected digit. Initial treatment with corticosteroid injection can be curative; however, because of the sustained synovial inflammation in the tendons, surgical treatment may be warranted.[8]

The most common flexor tendon to rupture is the FPL followed by the FDP to the index finger. This radial-to-ulnar pattern of flexor tendon rupture is opposite to the typical ulnar-to-radial direction of extensor tendon ruptures. Isolated tendon ruptures are more common than multiple tendon ruptures. The FPL is vulnerable to attritional damage as it crosses over the bony spicules at the scaphotrapezial joint, resulting in fraying of the tendon. Tenosynovitis of the tendon along with the attritional damage weakens the tendon, subsequently causing it to rupture.[8]

Rupture of the FPL occurring because of attritional damage over the scaphoid has been described as a Mannerfelt lesion.[37] FPL rupture leads to functional impairment of the thumb and necessitates surgical intervention to restore thumb function and prevent further tendon ruptures. Successful FPL reconstruction can be performed via an FDS tendon transfer, tendon graft using a palmaris longus or flexor carpi radialis, or an IP fusion.[8,27] Tendon transfers are useful in cases of long-standing tendon rupture and if the function of the musculotendinous unit is questionable. Tendon transfer can be combined with thumb IP joint fusion to regain satisfactory joint function. Ruptures of FDP tendons can be treated by transferring distal stump end to side of an adjacent digit's FDP tendon to perform an end-to-side repair.

## SUMMARY

A close working relationship between hand surgeons and rheumatologists is optimal to best treat patients with rheumatoid arthritis. Tendon rupture is a known risk with severe rheumatoid arthritis, especially with those patients who have not been treated with modern DMARDs. Recent advances in the medical management of rheumatoid patients may significantly decrease the rates of spontaneous tendon rupture in the future. In the meantime, tendon transfer remains the first-line treatment of tendon rupture. At the time of surgery, the underlying disorder causing the rupture should be addressed to prevent future ruptures. In the setting of an extensor tendon rupture, the dorsal synovitis and the subluxed and eroded distal ulna should be treated. Meanwhile, in the setting

of a flexor tendon rupture, the preexisting synovitis and bony spicules located over the scaphotrapezial joint should be debrided. Patients may present with multiple ruptures, often requiring multiple tendon transfers to regain function, and surgeons must always be prepared to encounter a larger number of involved tendons than the physical examination alone may suggest. Although not the first-line treatment, intercalated tendon grafting may be an option if the rupture is recent, the proximal musculotendinous unit shows adequate excursion, and there are no suitable tendons available for transfer.

## REFERENCES

1. Rasch EK, Hirsch R, Paulose-Ram R, et al. Prevalence of rheumatoid arthritis in persons 60 years of age and older in the United States: effect of different methods of case classification. Arthritis Rheum 2003;48(4):917–26.
2. Haugeberg G, Boyesen P, Helgetveit K, et al. Clinical and radiographic outcomes in patients diagnosed with early rheumatoid arthritis in the first years of the biologic treatment era: a 10-year prospective observational study. J Rheumatol 2015; 42(12):2279–87.
3. Herrinton LJ, Harrold L, Salman C, et al. Population variations in rheumatoid arthritis treatment and outcomes, Northern California, 1998-2009. Perm J 2016;20(1):4–12.
4. Gong HS, Lee JO, Baek GH, et al. Extensor tendon rupture in rheumatoid arthritis: a survey of patients between 2005 and 2010 at five Korean hospitals. Hand Surg 2012;17(1):43–7.
5. Chung US, Kim JH, Seo WS, et al. Tendon transfer or tendon graft for ruptured finger extensor tendons in rheumatoid hands. J Hand Surg Eur Vol 2010;35(4): 279–82.
6. Nalebuff EA. Present status of rheumatoid hand surgery. Am J Surg 1971;122(3):304–18.
7. Feldon P, Terrono AL, Nalebuff EA, et al. Rheumatoid arthritis and other connective tissue diseases. In: Wolfe SW, editor. Green's operative hand surgery, vol. 2. Philadelphia: Churchill Livingstone; 2011. p. 1993–2065.
8. Schindele SF, Herren DB, Simmen BR. Tendon reconstruction for the rheumatoid hand. Hand Clin 2011;27(1):105–13.
9. Malipeddi A, Reddy VR, Kallarackal G. Posterior interosseous nerve palsy: an unusual complication of rheumatoid arthritis: case report and review of the literature. Semin Arthritis Rheum 2011;40(6):576–9.
10. Magnell TD, Pochron MD, Condit DP. The intercalated tendon graft for treatment of extensor pollicis longus tendon rupture. J Hand Surg Am 1988; 13(1):105–9.

11. Nakamura S, Katsuki M. Tendon grafting for multiple extensor tendon ruptures of fingers in rheumatoid hands. J Hand Surg Br 2002;27(4):326–8.

12. Millender LH, Nalebuff EA, Albin R, et al. Dorsal tenosynovectomy and tendon transfer in the rheumatoid hand. J Bone Joint Surg Am 1974;56(3):601–10.

13. Bora FW Jr, Osterman AL, Thomas VJ, et al. The treatment of ruptures of multiple extensor tendons at wrist level by a free tendon graft in the rheumatoid patient. J Hand Surg Am 1987;12(6):1038–40.

14. Chu PJ, Lee HM, Hou YT, et al. Extensor-tendons reconstruction using autogenous palmaris longus tendon grafting for rheumatoid arthritis patients. J Orthop Surg Res 2008;3:16.

15. Garner RW, Mowat AG, Hazleman BL. Wound healing after operations of patients with rheumatoid arthritis. J Bone Joint Surg Br 1973;55(1):134–44.

16. Chetta MD, Ono S, Chung KC. Partial extensor carpi radialis longus turn-over tendon transfer for reconstruction of the extensor pollicis longus tendon in the rheumatoid hand: case report. J Hand Surg Am 2012;37(6):1217–20.

17. Browne EZ Jr, Teague MA, Snyder CC. Prevention of extensor lag after indicis proprius tendon transfer. J Hand Surg Am 1979;4(2):168–72.

18. Moore JR, Weiland AJ, Valdata L. Independent index extension after extensor indicis proprius transfer. J Hand Surg Am 1987;12(2):232–6.

19. Pulvertaft RG. Tendon grafts for flexor tendon injuries in the fingers and thumb; a study of technique and results. J Bone Joint Surg Br 1956;38-B(1):175–94.

20. Lubahn JD, Williams DP. Tendon transfers used for treatment of rheumatoid disorders. In: Weisel SW, editor. Operative techniques in orthopaedic surgery, vol. 3. Philadelphia: Lippincott Williams & Wilkins; 2011. p. 2608–18.

21. Ozalp T, Ozdemir O, Coskunol E, et al. Extensor indicis proprius transfers for extensor pollicis longus ruptures secondary to rheumatoid arthritis. Acta Orthop Traumatol Turc 2007;41(1):48–52 [in Turkish].

22. Backhouse KM. Abductor pollicis longus musculotendinous split as a replacement motor for ruptured extensor pollicis longus. Hand 1981;13(3):271–5.

23. Harrison S, Swannell AJ, Ansell BM. Repair of extensor pollicis longus using extensor pollicis brevis in rheumatoid arthritis. Ann Rheum Dis 1972;31(6):490–2.

24. Goodman SM, Menon I, Christos PJ, et al. Management of perioperative tumour necrosis factor alpha inhibitors in rheumatoid arthritis patients undergoing arthroplasty: a systematic review and meta-analysis. Rheumatology (Oxford) 2015;55(3):573–82.

25. Suzuki T, Iwamoto T, Ikegami H, et al. Comparison of surgical treatments for triple extensor tendon ruptures in rheumatoid hands: a retrospective study of 48 cases. Mod Rheumatol 2016;26(2):206–10.

26. Vaughan-Jackson OJ. Rupture of extensor tendons by attrition at the inferior radio-ulnar joint; report of two cases. J Bone Joint Surg Br 1948;30B(3):528–30.

27. Moore JR, Weiland AJ, Valdata L. Tendon ruptures in the rheumatoid hand: analysis of treatment and functional results in 60 patients. J Hand Surg Am 1987;12(1):9–14.

28. Sakuma Y, Ochi K, Iwamoto T, et al. Number of ruptured tendons and surgical delay as prognostic factors for the surgical repair of extensor tendon ruptures in the rheumatoid wrist. J Rheumatol 2014;41(2):265–9.

29. Boyes JM. Bunnell's surgery of the hand. 5th edition. Philadelphia: Lippincott; 1970.

30. Nalebuff EA, Patel MR. Flexor digitorum sublimis transfer for multiple extensor tendon ruptures in rheumatoid arthritis. Plast Reconstr Surg 1973;52(5):530–3.

31. Howell JW, Merritt WH, Robinson SJ. Immediate controlled active motion following zone 4-7 extensor tendon repair. J Hand Ther 2005;18(2):182–90.

32. Millis MB, Millender LH, Nalebuff EA. Stiffness of the proximal interphalangeal joints in rheumatoid arthritis. The role of flexor tenosynovitis. J Bone Joint Surg Am 1976;58(6):801–5.

33. Ertel AN, Millender LH, Nalebuff E, et al. Flexor tendon ruptures in patients with rheumatoid arthritis. J Hand Surg Am 1988;13(6):860–6.

34. Simmen BR, Kolling C, Herren DB. The management of the rheumatoid wrist. Curr Orthop 2007;21(5):344–57.

35. Barnes CG, Currey HL. Carpal tunnel syndrome in rheumatoid arthritis. A clinical and electrodiagnostic survey. Ann Rheum Dis 1967;26(3):226–33.

36. van der Heijde DM, van 't Hof MA, van Riel PL, et al. Judging disease activity in clinical practice in rheumatoid arthritis: first step in the development of a disease activity score. Ann Rheum Dis 1990;49(11):916–20.

37. Mannerfelt L, Norman O. Attrition ruptures of flexor tendons in rheumatoid arthritis caused by bony spurs in the carpal tunnel. A clinical and radiological study. J Bone Joint Surg Br 1969;51(2):270–7.

# Tendon Transfers for the Hypoplastic Thumb

Lindley B. Wall, MD*, Charles A. Goldfarb, MD

## KEYWORDS

- Hypoplastic thumb • Radial longtitudinal deficiency • Huber • Flexor digitorum superficialis
- Opposition transfer

## KEY POINTS

- Types 2 and 3A hypoplastic thumbs can be augmented by the Huber and flexor digitorum superficialis (FDS) opposition transfers.
- The Huber opposition transfer involves transfer of the abductor digiti minimi muscle from the ulnar side of the hand, improving opposition strength and thenar bulk.
- The FDS opposition transfer uses the FDS of the ring finger to transfer to the thumb metacarpophalangeal (MP) joint to improve opposition strength and can also be used to stabilize an unstable thumb MP joint.

## BACKGROUND

Thumb hypoplasia is a manifestation of radial longitudinal dysplasia, incomplete development of the radial or preaxial side of the upper extremity. Thumb hypoplasia describes underdevelopment of the thumb and its related structures. When treating individuals with thumb hypoplasia, the surgeon should always be aware of the potentially life-threatening associated conditions and syndromes; these include Fanconi anemia, Holt-Oram syndrome, VACTERL association, and thrombocytopenia absent radius syndrome. The authors recommend screening all individuals with thumb hypoplasia for these conditions by either referring the patient for a genetics consultation or obtaining a complete blood count, renal ultrasound, cardiac evaluation, spine radiograph, and consideration of chromosomal breakage test for Fanconi anemia. Once the screening has been completed, attention can turn to the hand for evaluation of thumb function.

Thumb hypoplasia was originally classified by Blauth[1] and subsequently modified by Buck-Gramko[2] and Manske and colleagues[3] (**Table 1**).

The classification system is dependent on the degree of hypoplasia, ranging from a slightly smaller thumb to a completely absent thumb. The modification proposed by Manske and colleagues[3] divides grade III based on the stability of the thumb carpometacarpal (CMC) joint. The modified classification provides surgeons guidance with regards to treatment of these underdeveloped thumbs. Although some surgeons may choose to reconstruct all forms of hypoplastic thumbs, most Western surgeons use the classification and reconstruct thumbs type II and IIIA and choose pollicization for grades IIIB, IV, and V thumbs.

When considering reconstruction for types II and IIIA, there are 3 specific components to be considered:

1. There is hypoplasia of the thumb muscles, intrinsics only in type II and extrinsic with intrinsic muscles in type 3.
2. There is instability of the thumb metacarpophalangeal (MP) joint. The MP joint instability must be addressed in order to provide stability for use and function of the thumb specifically with

Financial Disclosure: No commercial or financial conflicts to disclose.
Department of Orthopaedic Surgery, Washington University School of Medicine, 425 South Euclid Avenue, Suite 5505, St Louis, MO 63110, USA
* Corresponding author.
E-mail address: wallli@wudosis.wustl.edu

Hand Clin 32 (2016) 417–421
http://dx.doi.org/10.1016/j.hcl.2016.03.012
0749-0712/16/$ – see front matter © 2016 Elsevier Inc. All rights reserved.

hand.theclinics.com

| Table 1 |
| :--- |
| **Thumb Hypoplasia Blauth Classification, modified by Manske** |

| Hypoplastic Thumb Classification | |
| :--- | :--- |
| Type 1 | Slightly small thumb |
| Type 2 | Small thumb with<br>• Narrow first web space<br>• Unstable metacarpophalangeal joint<br>• Deficient thenar musculature |
| Type 3a | Type II with<br>• Extrinsic tendon abnormalities<br>• Metacarpal hypoplasia<br>• Stable CMC joint |
| Type 3b | Type II with<br>• Extrinsic tendon abnormalities<br>• Absent metacarpal base/CMC instability |
| Type 4 | Floating thumb |
| Type 5 | Absent thumb |

regards to pinch and grasp. This instability can be isolated to laxity of the ulnar collateral ligament or can be a global instability.

3. The first web space may be narrowed, requiring widening with a Z-plasty or dorsal transposition flap. This widening can be challenging to recognize in small hands, and as a guide, in a normal hand the distance between the thumb and index metacarpal head should be the same as that of the index to small metacarpal head.

There are 2 commonly used tendon transfers to augment thumb function and strength in opposition: the Huber opposition transfer[4–13] and the flexor digitorum superficialis (FDS) opposition transfer.[11–16] Both techniques are effective in improving thumb function, and each has specific advantages.

The Huber opposition transfer involves transfer of the abductor digiti minimi (ADM) muscle from the ulnar border of the hand to the thumb. This muscle is a reliable transfer candidate; it is always present in radial longitudinal deficiency, and there is little (if any) notable deficit once transferred. The ADM is rotated across the palm, augments thumb opposition, and increases bulk in the thenar region, improving cosmesis of the hand. Also, the transfer does not require the use of a pulley, which the FDS transfer necessitates. Unfortunately, the muscle is short and has a very small tendon insertion. As a result, this muscle cannot be used to help stabilize the thumb MP joint. Additional steps, such as imbrication of the ulnar collateral ligament and capsule of the MP joint, must be performed to create stability of this joint. This step is important because the

pull of the Huber transfer on the APB insertion adds a further deforming force to the UCL and can worsen UCL instability if this is not addressed. Last, the authors do not use the Huber in older children because the authors have been limited in the length of the transfer, although the necessary length has not been quantified at this time.

The FDS opposition transfer is the alternative to the Huber to improve hypoplastic thumb strength and function. This technique uses a flexor tendon from one of the ulnar digits, typically the ring finger or long finger, as a transfer to augment thumb strength. As with the ADM, the FDS is present in the ring finger and can be reliably harvested. There has been no documentation of decreased strength in the hand with this transfer. The FDS passes across the palm to the thumb. This technique does not augment the thenar eminence cosmetically, but the tendon length is beneficial because it allows for simultaneous reconstruction of the collateral ligament of the thumb MP joint.

## SURGICAL TECHNIQUES
### Huber Opposition Transfer

A curvilinear incision is made along the ulnar border of the hand, at or slightly volar to the glabrous, nonglaborous border. This incision extends from the pisiform ending just proximal to the MP flexion crease of the small finger (**Fig. 1**). The palmar skin

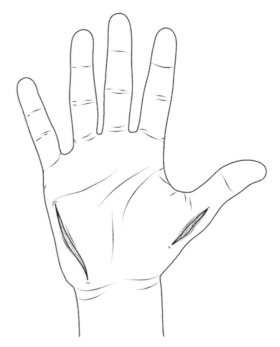

**Fig. 1.** The incisions for the Huber opposition transfer. A curvilinear incision is made along the ulnar boarder of the hand, and a second incision is placed over the radial boarder of the thumb MP joint.

is elevated exposing the underlying musculature. The ADM muscle is identified and isolated. There are 2 tendinous insertions, which are isolated and detached distally. The ADM is then mobilized proximally to its origin on the pisiform. Care is taken to protect the neurovascular bundle that is entering the muscle deep and radial, near the pisiform origin. A blunt Kelly clamp is used to create a generous subcutaneous tunnel from the level of the pisiform to the radial border of the thumb MP joint. A longitudinal incision is made over the radial aspect of the thumb MP joint to accept the transfer. The ADM is folded, like turning the page of a book, across the palm, and is then passed through this large subcutaneous tunnel to the thumb (**Fig. 2**). If length as needed, the origin of the ADM can be detached from the ulnar border of the pisiform, allowing further length to reach across the palm. The ulnar incision is irrigated and closed. The tendon of the ADM is then sutured to residual abductor pollicis brevis tendon, the joint capsule, and radial collateral ligament of the thumb MP joint. If there is instability to the thumb MP joint ulnarly, a counterincision is made and the joint capsule is imbricated or ligament reconstruction is performed.

## Flexor Digitorum Superficialis Opposition Transfer

A longitudinal (or transverse) incision is made just proximal to the MP flexion crease of the ring finger,

approximately 1.5 cm in length (**Fig. 3**). The A1 pulley is opened, and the FDS tendon is identified. It is drawn out of the incision and transected as distally as possible. It is not necessary to incise further in the digit for additional length because the tendon length obtained from an incision at the level of the A1 pulley is adequate for the transfer. A second incision is made proximal to the wrist flexion crease and slightly ulnar to the palmaris longus tendon, approximately 2 cm in length. The FDS tendon to the ring finger is identified in the volar wrist wound. Often it is necessary to free the tendon from surrounding adhesions in the distal wound to allow it to be drawn out in the proximal wound. The distal incision is then closed. The FDS must now be taken across the palm to the thumb MP joint (**Fig. 4**). There are multiple options for creation of a pulley to provide an effective line of pull for the FDS tendon,[17] and no one pulley has been found to be superior. More distally placed pulleys will result in greater flexion and adduction force of the transfer, whereas more proximal pulleys result in greater palmar abduction of the transfer. The authors recommend using the flexor carpi ulnaris (FCU) tendon as a pulley. A small portion of the FCU tendon is cut, folded,

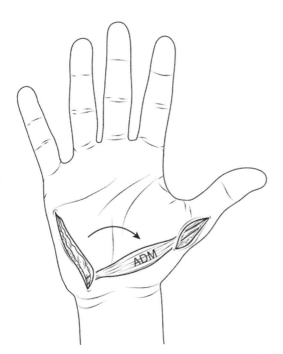

**Fig. 2.** The ADM muscle is transferred across the palm to the thumb MP joint, passed subcutaneously.

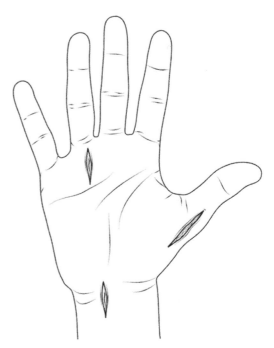

**Fig. 3.** The incisions for the FDS opposition transfer. One incision is made at the base of the ring finger for harvest of the FDS tendon. A second incision is made proximal to the wrist flexion crease to bring out the FDS tendon and placed through the FCU tendon. A third incision is made over the radial boarder of the thumb MP joint.

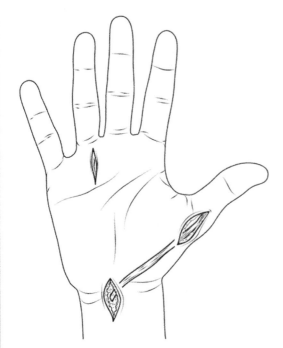

**Fig. 4.** The FDS tendon is transferred across the palm to the thumb MP joint, passed subcutaneously.

and sutured in place as a tendon loop, to act as a pulley. Another option is to simply pass the FDS tendon through the FCU tendon with a stay stitch placed proximally to avoid proximal migration of the incision in the FCU. An alternative is to use the transverse carpal ligament as a pulley. A strip of tissue can be used from the ligament to create a pulley.

After the chosen pulley is created, a blunt Kelly retractor is passed across the palm, making a wide tunnel through which the FDS tendon is passed. The proximal incisions are closed. An accepting incision is made on the radial border of the thumb MP joint, and the FDS tendon is delivered. A hole is created transversely through the neck of the metacarpal. This hole can be made with a drill or a manual punch tool. The FDS tendon is passed to the ulnar side of the thumb MP joint. The tendon is secured to the palmarly abducted metacarpal. The thumb ulnar collateral ligament is reconstructed by suturing to the periosteum at the base of the proximal phalanx (or attaching with a suture anchor). If there is instability of the radial collateral ligament of the thumb MP joint, the FDS tendon can be split longitudinally, with half passed into the metacarpal to reconstruct the ulnar collateral ligament and the remaining half used on the radial side to reconstruct the radial collateral ligament.

## General Technical Considerations

As with all tendon transfer procedures, the authors recommend closing the incisions as one proceeds through the case; this prevents the need to close multiple incisions after the transfer has been sutured, risking loosening. When considering the appropriate tightness of the transfer, the authors recommend tensioning the thumb out of the plane of the fingers and into palmar abduction with the wrist in a neutral position. Care is taken not to strangulate the pedicle of the ADM muscle belly with a narrow tunnel. The authors have found that there is risk of vascular compromise with overtightening the ADM transfer, and the transferred muscle can exert compression at the carpal tunnel.[18] Last, some surgeons may choose to place a 0.045 or 0.035 Kirschner wire to hold the thumb opposed to decrease stress and tension on the transferred during the time of healing.

The authors' postoperative protocol for both of these transfers includes a long-arm cast for the younger children, up to approximately age 7, and short arm cast for older children. The authors recommend immobilization for 5 weeks while the transfers heal. After 5 weeks, the cast and pins are removed; a splint is made by the therapist, and gentle motion is started. This removable orthoplast, thumb spica forearm-based splint is used for the next 4 weeks at all times except for monitored range-of-motion exercises. At approximately 9 to 10 weeks, the authors transition out of the brace during the day for normal activities and continue wearing the brace at night for one additional month. At this point, gentle strengthening is started.

## OUTCOMES

Currently, there is minimal literature concerning the outcomes of opposition transfers for the hypoplastic thumb. At this time, there are no reports of the outcomes of the Huber opposition transfer. Two studies have reported outcomes of the FDS opposition transfer for types II and IIIA hypoplastic thumbs.[19,20] De Kraker and colleagues[19] assessed 27 thumbs, 21 that had undergone tendon transfer and 6 that were treated nonoperatively. They found that the FDS transfer significantly improved strength in those that had undergone surgery and that strength (grip and pinch) was 50% and 35% of normal in type II and IIIA, respectively. Vuillermin and colleagues[20] reported on 40 thumbs at a minimum 2-years follow-up and found grip and pinch strength was approximately 50% of normal and that overall perceived function and happiness were high. There was no difference between the different pulleys used, and 36 of the thumbs underwent UCL reconstruction. Both studies reported increased stability of the thumb MP joints after reconstruction.

Quantitative assessment of outcomes is difficult to perform secondary to the varying levels of hypoplasia and severity of involvement. In addition, as with most congenital hand procedures, the progressing age of the child makes both subjective and objective outcome assessments difficult to compare. However, there are numerous studies reporting specific surgical techniques for opposition reconstruction, and the authors' preference for reconstruction is described here.

## REFERENCES

1. Blauth W. Numerical variations. In: Schneider-Sickert F, editor. Congential variations of the hand. Berlin: Springer Science & Business Media; 1981. p. 120–1.

2. Buck-Gramcko D. Congenital malformations of the hand and forearm. Chir Main 2002;21(2):70–101.

3. Manske PR, McCarroll HR Jr, James M. Type III—a hypoplastic thumb. J Hand Surg Am 1995;20(2):246–53.

4. Manske PR, McCarroll HR. Abductor digiti minimi opponensplasty in congenital radial dysplasia. J Hand Surg Am 1978;3(6):552–9.

5. Huber E. Hilfsoperation bei Medianuslähmung. Dtsch Z Chir 1921;162(3–4):271–5.

6. Littler JW, Cooley SG. Opposition of the thumb and its restoration by abductor digiti quinti transfer. J Bone Joint Surg Am 1963;45:1389–96.

7. Ogino T, Minami A, Fukuda K. Abductor digiti minimi opponensplasty in hypoplastic thumb. J Hand Surg Br 1986;11(3):372–7.

8. Ishida O, Ikuta Y, Sunagawa T, et al. Abductor digiti minimi musculocutaneous island flap as an opposition transfer: a case report. J Hand Surg Am 2003;28(1):130–2.

9. Upton J, Taghinia AH. Abductor digiti minimi myocutaneous flap for opponensplasty in congenital hypoplastic thumbs. Plast Reconstr Surg 2008;122(6):1807–11.

10. de Roode CP, James MA, McCarroll HR Jr. Abductor digit minimi opponensplasty: technique, modifications, and measurement of opposition. Tech Hand Up Extrem Surg 2010;14(1):51–3.

11. Hostin R, James MA. Reconstruction of the hypoplastic thumb. J Am Soc Surg Hand 2004;4(4):275–90.

12. McDonald TJ, James MA, McCarroll HR Jr, et al. Reconstruction of the type IIIA hypoplastic thumb. Tech Hand Up Extrem Surg 2008;2:79–84.

13. Light T, Gaffey J. Reconstruction of the hypoplastic thumb. J Hand Surg 2010;35A:474–9.

14. Christen T, Dautel G. Type II and IIIA thumb hypoplasia reconstruction. J Hand Surg Am 2013;38(10):2009–15.

15. Kozin SH, Ezaki M. Flexor digitorum superficialis opponensplasty with ulnar collateral ligament reconstruction for thumb deficiency. Tech Hand Up Extrem Surg 2010;14(1):46–50.

16. Smith P, Sivakumar B, Hall R, et al. Blauth II thumb hypoplasia: a management algorithm for the unstable metacarpophalangeal joint. J Hand Surg Eur Vol 2012;37(8):745–50.

17. Lee DH, Oakes JE, Birmingham AL, et al. Tendon transfers for thumb opposition: a biomechanical study of pulley location and two insertion sites. J Hand Surg Am 2003;28(6):1002–8.

18. Goldfarb CA, Leversedge FJ, Manske PR. Bilateral carpal tunnel syndrome after abductor digiti minimi opposition transfer: a case report. J Hand Surg Am 2003;28(4):681–4.

19. De Kraker M, Delles RW, Zuidam JM, et al. Outcome of flexor digitorum superficialis opponensplasty for type II and IIIA thumb hypoplasia. J Hand Surg Eur Vol 2016;41(3):258–64.

20. Vuillermin C, Butler L, Lake A, et al. Flexor digitorum superficialis opposition transfer for augmenting function in types II and IIIA thumb hypoplasia. J Hand Surg Am 2016;41(2):244–9.

# Cerebral Palsy Tendon Transfers

## Flexor Carpi Ulnaris to Extensor Carpi Radialis Brevis and Extensor Pollicis Longus Reroutement

Anchal Bansal, BS, Lindley B. Wall, MD,
Charles A. Goldfarb, MD*

**KEYWORDS**

- Cerebral palsy • EPL tendon reroutement • FCU tendon transfer

**KEY POINTS**

- Children with spastic hemiplegic cerebral palsy may benefit from tendon transfer surgery if therapy is not successful in addressing functional and esthetic limitations.
- A position of wrist and thumb flexion is common and limits grasp and overall function. If the fingers can still be extended in a wrist neutral posture, the patient may be a good candidate for surgery.
- Transfer of the flexor carpi ulnaris to the extensor carpi radialis brevis is a commonly performed and reliable surgery to allow a neutral wrist posture and improved function and appearance.
- A thumb-in-palm deformity limits function including large object grasp and finger flexion and can be helped with an extensor pollicis longus reroutement along with a thenar release.

## INTRODUCTION: NATURE OF THE PROBLEM

Cerebral palsy (CP), a static condition typically related to a perinatal cerebral insult, is the most common motor disability in childhood. Although the neurologic damage is nonprogressive, the motor disability and physical deformity often worsen over time as a result of abnormal muscle tone and firing patterns and growth leading to joint contractures, postural imbalance, and selective disuse.[1] Of children with CP, 81% have the spastic subtype that is characterized by varying degrees of muscular hypertonicity and is most amenable to surgical intervention.[2]

Common upper extremity manifestations include pronation of the forearm, flexion and ulnar deviation of the wrist, and adduction and flexion

of the thumb, causing a thumb-in-palm deformity (**Fig. 1**). The wrist and thumb deformities may impair both grasp and release as well as lateral pinch, leading to difficulties with daily activities and, if severe, difficulties with hygiene. Furthermore, esthetic concerns may affect the child's psyche, self-esteem, and social development.[3]

There are several well-accepted upper extremity surgeries that have been demonstrated to have a positive impact on both upper extremity function and appearance for children with CP.[4] This article focuses on 2 such transfers: the flexor carpi ulnaris (FCU) to extensor carpi radialis brevis (ECRB) transfer[5,6] (also known as the Green transfer) for the wrist and thenar release combined with rerouting of the extensor pollicis longus (EPL) tendon[7–9] for the thumb.

Financial Disclosure: No commercial or financial conflicts to disclose.
Washington University School of Medicine, 660 South Euclid Avenue, St Louis, MO 63110, USA
* Corresponding author.
E-mail address: goldfarbc@wudosis.wustl.edu

Hand Clin 32 (2016) 423–430
http://dx.doi.org/10.1016/j.hcl.2016.03.010
0749-0712/16/$ – see front matter © 2016 Elsevier Inc. All rights reserved.

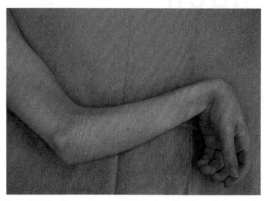

**Fig. 1.** Classic resting position in CP. The elbow is in flexion, the forearm in pronation, and the wrist is flexed. In this patient, with the wrist flexed, the thumb is in a reasonable resting position. The thumb is examined when the wrist is maximally flexed to determine if there is a thumb-in-palm deformity. (*Courtesy of* Charles A. Goldfarb, MD).

## PREOPERATIVE PLANNING—FLEXOR CARPI ULNARIS TO EXTENSOR CARPI RADIALIS BREVIS TENDON TRANSFER

This transfer removes a deforming force (FCU) causing wrist flexion and ulnar deviation while concurrently augmenting the weaker dorsiflexion and supination forces.[5,6,10]

### Patient Selection

Careful patient selection helps to assure success and functional improvement. Numerous factors have been implicated in influencing the outcomes of the transfer: cognitive function, hand sensibility (stereognosis), patient age, caretaker involvement, degree of voluntary motor control, amount of attention paid to the extremity, and phasic muscle activity.

### Type of Cerebral Palsy

Patients with spastic hemiplegia may gain the most from surgery, because the affected hand is primarily used to assist the normal hand in performing daily tasks. Incremental unilateral improvements can significantly enhance the child's bimanual capability and overall quality of life.[11]

Grasp and release pattern is a critical factor affecting patient outcome. Patients resting in wrist flexion have a difficult timing making a tight fist; a surgery to extend the wrist to a neutral posture can help improve grasp. It is important to note, however, that some patients rely on the tenodesis effect and use wrist flexion to extend the fingers and "release." Therefore, during preoperative

assessment, the surgeon or therapist must assure that extending the wrist does not compromise the ability to open and close the fingers (Zancolli testing[12] of finger tightness with wrist extension). An FCU to extensor digitorum transfer may be considered in patients who cannot extend the fingers with the wrist in neutral, becasue it augments digital extension and is less likely to result in excessively strong wrist extension.[13]

The authors hesitate to perform the FCU-to-ECRB transfer when the wrist lacks 45° (or more) of extension with the fingers straight. In the younger patient, the finger flexors may be lengthened at the time of the tendon transfer surgery. In older patients, a wrist fusion with proximal row carpectomy (PRC) can provide a stable, functional wrist with improved finger motion through shortening the bony structure via the PRC.

### Age

The importance of age is debated in the literature. Some argue that postponing surgery until the patient is mentally and physically mature limits complications resulting from future growth and unreliable adherence to postoperative care and therapy. One study[14] reported complications, including extension deformity, supination deformity, and flexion recurrence, in 82% of children younger than 13 years compared with a 25% rate in the older children. Furthermore, the younger group comprised 75% (9/12) of the total population developing complications. Others maintain that surgery at a younger age, less than 8 years, allows more seamless utilization of the corrected hand, because children have not adapted to single-handedness or begun to ignore the disabled hand. Furthermore, early deformity correction may preempt the emergence of contractures and limit joint developmental anomalies,[3] and greater skeletal flexibility may permit children to progress through physical therapy more easily than adults. Psychological factors should also be considered. Early surgical intervention, before school age, limits the social stigmatization and physical obstacles faced by these children. Despite the controversy, it is generally agreed that surgery should be deferred at least until children are old enough to understand the nature of surgery and participate in rehabilitation; this is generally reported as being at least 4 to 6 years of age.[5,13–15]

### Cognition and Motivation

Cognitive function and motivation are important prerequisites for the patient to participate in therapy and make functional use of the hand. Differing opinions exist as to the role of formal IQ testing.

When it has been applied, an IQ of 70 to 80 has generally been reported as the minimum threshold of required intelligence, below which worse outcomes are noted.[5,16] Alternatively, adequate intelligence can be determined through indirect cognitive testing focusing on task performance, interaction, school reports, and overall daily functioning.[13] Motivation is a more abstract concept and must be judged by both surgeons and therapists. Patients who do not consistently follow the rehabilitation protocol have worse outcomes than those who adhere; this is particularly important in patients with lower cognitive functioning.[17] In these individuals, motivation and family discipline are the most predictive factors for successful rehabilitation.[5]

## Preoperative Function (Strength, Voluntary Control, Phasic Contraction)

No uniform recommendation exists for the amount of hand function required before surgery. However, a greater degree of active preoperative hand usage portends better postoperative outcomes.[18] One study reported this as the most important prognostic factor for surgical success with a significantly greater rate of improvement (80%) among patients demonstrating assistive activity of the affected hand compared with patients without functional use (50%).[15] Tendon transfer surgery is contraindicated in patients presenting with fixed flexion deformities or a lack of voluntary motor control in the hand.[1,5] Fixed flexion deformities must be addressed and the patient reassessed before tendon transfer is considered.[5] Furthermore, the FCU must have adequate tone and strength for the transfer to be effective. The phase of muscle firing may also be evaluated[19,20] by dynamic electromyography testing but is not imperative. The best results are reported when FCU and ECRB operate in the same phase.[1,10,19–21]

## Sensibility

Improved hand sensibility is also associated with better postoperative results, possibly because the level of tactile sensation influences patterns of hand usage.[1,5,11,13,16] In fact, Green and Banks[5] originally discussed it as one of the most important determinants of surgical outcome.

## PREOPERATIVE PLANNING—EXTENSOR POLLICIS LONGUS REROUTING AND THENAR RELEASE
### Patient Selection

The thumb-in-palm deformity impedes pinch, grasp, and release functions and blocks finger flexion by occupying space in the palm. Furthermore, limited thumb extension and first web space contracture prevent the child from handling larger objects.

EPL rerouting is indicated for correction of thumb-in-palm deformity as characterized by the following features:

1. Thumb rests in the palm with limited active extension; this limits function via the thumb position but also blocks finger flexion.
2. Thumb becomes tightly clenched within the fist when digits are flexed.
3. Ability of the patient to voluntarily control and use the extremity is intact but overall functionality is hindered by the deformity.[7]

The modified House classification of thumb deformity described by Tonkin and colleagues[22,23] may be used to assist with thumb assessment, but the guiding principle is to weaken spastic intrinsic muscles and supplement extension. Typically, a thenar slide and adductor release are used to weaken the intrinsic muscles and an EPL rerouting procedure is used together in most types of thumb-in-palm deformity, although those patients with flexor pollicis longus tightness require FPL lengthening as well.[24,25]

The primary patient factors to consider are similar to those listed above for the FCU-to-ECRB tendon transfer. A 2005 *Cochrane Review*[26] found little consensus on the relative impact of these factors and considerable methodological variability between studies. If the sole intent is addressing esthetic or hygienic concerns, successful surgery is possible in all patients, regardless of the above characteristics.[22,25,27]

## Age

Existing debate regarding early versus late surgery is again similar to that described for the FCU-to-ECRB tendon transfer. However, age has not been reported to negatively affect outcomes.[7,8,22] Importantly, the child should be old enough to participate in rehabilitation, and the minimum age range in the literature is 4 to 10 years.[1,7,8,22,25]

The following are contraindications to the procedure[22,25]:

1. Mental impairment severe enough to prevent participation in rehabilitation.
2. Lack of voluntary control over the EPL.
3. Primarily dystonic CP or extrapyramidal disease.

## SURGICAL TECHNIQUE—FLEXOR CARPI ULNARIS TO EXTENSOR CARPI RADIALIS BREVIS TENDON TRANSFER
### Preparation and Patient Positioning

After administration of general anesthesia, the patient is positioned supine with the arm extended on an arm table, sterilely prepared, and draped. The hand and forearm are exsanguinated and a non-sterile arm tourniquet is elevated.

### Surgical Approach

A longitudinal volar, ulnar incision begins at the wrist flexor crease and extends proximally at least 60% of the length of the forearm to expose the FCU.

### Surgical Procedure

Step 1 (**Fig. 2**):
- Identify the FCU tendon from its insertion on the pisiform to the proximal forearm.
- Identify and protect the ulnar nerve and artery, just deep and radial to the tendon.

Step 2 (**Fig. 3**):
- Divide the FCU at the pisiform, tag the tendon with suture, and dissect proximally.

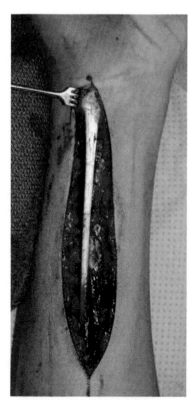

**Fig. 2.** Surgical incision and exposure of FCU tendon. (*Courtesy of* Charles A. Goldfarb, MD).

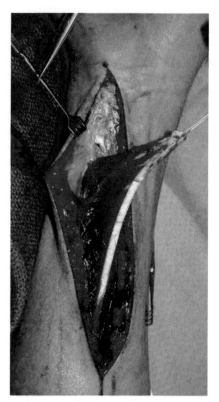

**Fig. 3.** Dissection of FCU with muscle detached from the ulna and the intermuscular septum. (*Courtesy of* Charles A. Goldfarb, MD).

- Remove attachments to the ulna and inter-muscular septum.
- Distal muscle (which is denervated from the procedure) can be excised to ease the passage and gliding of the tendon transfer.
- Preserve the muscle's proximal neurovascular pedicle.

Notably, a greater extent of proximal dissection confers a straighter line of tendon transfer pull and a larger supinator force. Release of the distal two-thirds of FCU has been shown to provide an additional 54° of supination when compared with release of the distal one-third alone.[5,17]

Step 3:
- Make a second, 3-cm longitudinal incision dorsally, just proximal to Lister tubercle over the second compartment to expose the ECRB and extensor carpi radialis longus (ECRL) tendons.
- Pass a large clamp from the dorsal incision, around the ulnar border of the ulna to the proximal aspect of the volar incision. This step is important because it creates the path of the transfer and, as such, a longitudinal course is optimal. The opening in the septum

is approximately 5 cm in length; the length is necessary to avoid constriction of the transfer.

Step 4 (**Fig. 4**):

- Most commonly the ECRB, rather than the ECRL, is used as the insertion site given its central insertion and, therefore, a more pure dorsiflexion force.
- Pass the FCU tendon and close the volar incision before suturing the transfer.
- Tension the wrist in the range of neutral to 10° of flexion[1,4,10,14,15,28] and weave the FCU into the desired extensor tendon using the Pulvertaft technique.[1]

Step 5:

- Deflate the tourniquet, obtain hemostasis, and close the dorsal wound.

### Immediate Postoperative Care

The extremity is lightly dressed and immobilized in a long arm bivalved cast with the wrist positioned at neutral, the forearm in maximal comfortable supination, and the elbow in near full extension (these positions are determined in part by additional surgeries). The bivalved cast accommodates swelling. CP patients are especially vulnerable to compartment syndrome because their altered tactile sensation may preclude early detection.

## REHABILITATION AND RECOVERY

Five weeks postoperatively[29]:

- A short arm, volar, removable splint is made with wrist in neutral. This splint is worn at all

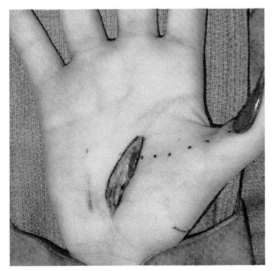

**Fig. 4.** Incision along the thenar crease for the thenar slide and adductor release.

times except during supervised exercises. Passive wrist flexion is avoided.

- Begin gentle active and passive wrist extension and forearm supination exercises/activities and progress to passive range of motion (except flexion).

Eight weeks postoperatively:

- Discontinue daytime splinting and continue nighttime splinting for a total of 12 weeks after surgery.
- Begin active wrist flexion exercises.
- Light, functional activities allowed.
- Begin progressive strengthening for wrist extension.

## SURGICAL TECHNIQUE—EXTENSOR POLLICIS LONGUS RE-REROUTING AND ABDUCTOR POLLICUS LONGUS RELEASE

### Surgical Approach

Three incisions are used with a single volar incision along the thenar crease for the adductor release. A dorsal incision over the thumb metacarpal and another incision adjacent to Lister tubercle facilitate the EPL rerouting.

### Surgical Procedure

Step 1 (see **Fig. 4**):

- A curved palmar incision along the thenar crease provides exposure.[8,23]
- The thenar muscles are identified and gently teased off the transverse carpal ligament (primarily the flexor pollicis brevis).
- The radial digital neurovascular bundle of the index finger is protected.
- The transverse carpal ligament is incised, and the contents of the carpal tunnel are retracted gently in an ulnar direction.
- The adductor pollicis is identified, taking care to protect the deep branches of the ulnar nerve and artery passing between the oblique and transverse heads.
- Release the transverse head from its origin on the palmar base of the third metacarpal and the oblique head from its origins on the capitate and palmar bases of the second and third metacarpals.[8,25]
- The wound is irrigated and closed.

Step 2:

- A longitudinal dorsal incision is made over the first metacarpal.
- The tight first dorsal interosseous muscle is released.
- The EPL tendon is identified distally in the wound and released just proximal to the extensor expansion at the metacarpophalangeal (MCP) joint.

**Step 3:**

- A 3-cm longitudinal incision is created over the dorsal, distal radius, just ulnar to Lister tubercle.
- The distally transected EPL is brought out of this incision.

**Step 4:**

- A small, curved clamp is passed from the distal incision, adjacent to the first dorsal compartment to exit in the proximal incision. Ideally the clamp passes through the compartment, but the goal is to simply hold the re-routed tendon in this more radial position; this can be accomplished without entirely passing through the compartment.
- The first dorsal compartment acts as a pulley, changing the EPL's vector of pull from ulnar to radial, and its action from extension adduction to extension abduction.
- The tendon is passed distally.
- The proximal wound is closed.

**Step 5:**

- If sufficient periosteum exists dorsally on the metacarpal, the EPL is passed beneath the periosteum and sutured to the periosteum to allow maximum extension force to the metacarpal. The tendon is then also reattached to its distal stump at the extensor expansion. Inevitably, some extra tendon is excised.
- Tension the EPL to a resting position of retropulsion (abduction and extension) when the wrist is in flexion. The thumb should rest in a more comfortable position adjacent to the index ray when the wrist is extended.
- Close the distal incision.
- A thumb spica cast is applied, which may be short- or long-armed depending on the age of the patient and the concurrent surgeries performed. The interphalangeal(IP) joint is included, and the thumb is held in midpalmar and radial abduction. MCP joint hyperextension is avoided.

## REHABILITATION AND RECOVERY— EXTENSOR POLLICIS LONGUS REROUTING AND THENAR RELEASE

Five weeks postoperatively[29]:

- A volar forearm thumb splint is fabricated to place the wrist in 15° extension and thumb in radial abduction (avoid MCP and IP joint hyperextension).
- Splint is worn at all times except during supervised exercises.
- Begin gentle active thumb extension/abduction exercises/activities and progress

to passive thumb extension/abduction as tolerated. Avoid passive thumb flexion.

Eight weeks postoperatively:

- Possible discontinuation of daytime splinting; nighttime splinting is continued for 3 months.
- Begin active thumb flexion/opposition exercises.
- Light, functional activities allowed with involved extremity.
- Initiate progressive thumb strengthening for extension or abduction.

## CLINICAL RESULTS

Part of the difficulty in comparing results between studies is the breadth of evaluation tools[26] and the lack of any standardization between them. The validity of these tools in accurately assessing improvement after surgical intervention is also a matter of debate, especially given the numerous child-centered variables in those with CP.[4,30] In addition, most children undergo multiple concurrent surgeries, further obscuring the measureable impact of any individual procedure.[9]

### Flexor Carpi Ulnaris to Extensor Carpi Radialis Brevis Transfer

The FCU-to-ECRB transfer is considered a key procedure for children with wrist flexion posture in CP with overall positive outcomes observed in appropriately selected patients (as long as the tendon transfer is not sutured in too much tension). Van Heest and colleagues[18] reported 2.5 levels of functional improvement based on the House scale following the procedure and noted this to be statistically similar to the outcomes observed after brachioradialis and ECU transfers. Roth and colleagues[11] observed that, although total range of motion was unchanged with surgery, wrist extension improved by 53° due to shifting of the center of the arc of motion from a flexed position to a neutral position. Other investigators have reached similar conclusions for both wrist flexion and forearm supination.[13,15] Finally, the reported incidence of postoperative, undesired extension deformities ranges from 13% to 69%.[13,16,19] Patterson and colleagues[14] reported that patients demonstrated good wrist positioning until the development of extension deformity, which arose approximately 38 months after initial surgery. These deformities were far more prevalent in patients younger than 13 years compared with the older population. Strategies to decrease this risk include avoiding overcorrecting or prolonged casting, especially in young patients, and intensive stretching and therapy protocols.[1,9,14] Treatment is challenging and the patient may be best managed with lengthening of the wrist extensor or takedown and reinsertion of the transfer. However, in an older child with a marked extension position, a wrist fusion is the most straightforward and reliable intervention.

### Extensor Pollicis Longus Rerouting and Thenar Release

A *Cochrane Review*[26] concluded modest overall gains with surgery but found it difficult to meaningfully compare results between studies. All included studies reported that in most patients the thumb remained out of the palm at follow-up. One study found that MCP abduction range increased by 19° after an average of 3 to 4 operations, including EPL rerouting and thenar release. Although this was not enough to change patients from dependent to independent functional status, it was sufficient to maintain the thumb out of the palm in 29 of 32 patients, thus significantly improving their quality of life. Furthermore, 26 of 32 patients gained lateral pinch function.[23] Another study reported that postsurgical first web space angles greater than 45°, and functional improvements were observed in 12 of 14 of their patients.[27] Several investigators have noted wider grip, larger object handling, and bimanual task completion including eating and dressing, to be the most frequently improved functions.[7,27,31] Range of motion on physical examination should not be used as an indicator for surgical need or to assess its success, because it correlates poorly with activity measures and dynamic range of motion during functional performance. Validated activity measures are better, although still imperfect, assessment aids.[4,30] Hyperextension instability of the MCP joint is an observed complication resulting from augmentation of muscles acting distal to this joint, leading to an adduction instead of abduction moment acting on the thumb metacarpal. It can be prevented by performing MCP joint capsulodesis or arthrodesis at the time of surgery in those patients deemed at risk.[9,23,27,32]

### SUMMARY

Surgical intervention in appropriately selected CP patients results in better functional outcomes compared with nonsurgical interventions, including physical therapy, splinting, and botulinum injections.[4,9] However, patients must be carefully chosen with regard to their specific deformities, overall health status, goals of surgery, and ability to appropriately rehabilitate because amount of expected improvement is heavily dependent on these variables. Furthermore, current assessment measures

may not accurately reflect functional impairment, and a child's test performance is impacted by several variables including emotional state, task familiarity, and personnel present during examination. Therefore, repeated multidisciplinary assessments using several evaluation methods are vital for gaining accurate knowledge of physical ability. Finally, routine participation in intensive postoperative physical and occupational therapy both at home and in a formal setting is ideal for achieving optimal outcomes.

### REFERENCES

1. de Roode CP, James MA, Van Heest AE. Tendon transfers and releases for the forearm, wrist, and hand in spastic hemiplegic cerebral palsy. Tech Hand Up Extrem Surg 2010;14(2): 129–34.
2. CDC. Data and statistics | cerebral palsy | NCBDDD | CDC. [Internet]. Available at: http://www.cdc.gov/ncbddd/cp/data.html. Accessed January 22, 2016.
3. Leafblad ND, Van Heest AE. Management of the spastic wrist and hand in cerebral palsy. J Hand Surg Am 2015;40(5):1035–40.
4. Van Heest AE, Bagley A, Molitor F, et al. Tendon transfer surgery in upper-extremity cerebral palsy is more effective than botulinum toxin injections or regular, ongoing therapy. J Bone Joint Surg Am 2015;97(7):529–36.
5. Green WT, Banks HH. Flexor carpi ulnaris transplant and its use in cerebral palsy. J Bone Joint Surg Am 1962;44(7):1343–430.
6. Green WT, McDermott LJ. Operative treatment of cerebral palsy of spastic type. J Am Med Assoc 1942;118(6):434–40.
7. Manske PR. Redirection of extensor pollicis longus in the treatment of spastic thumb-in-palm deformity. J Hand Surg Am 1985;10(4):553–60.
8. Matev IB. Surgical treatment of flexion-adduction contracture of the thumb in cerebral palsy. Acta Orthop Scand 1970;41(4):439–45.
9. Smitherman JA, Davids JR, Tanner S, et al. Functional outcomes following single-event multi-level surgery of the upper extremity for children with hemiplegic cerebral palsy. J Bone Joint Surg Am 2011;93(7):655–61.
10. Manske PR. Cerebral palsy of the upper extremity. Hand Clin 1990;6(4):697–709.
11. Roth JH, O'Grady SE, Richards RS, et al. Functional outcome of upper limp tendon transfers performed in children with spastic hemiplegia. J Hand Surg Br 1993;18(3):299–303.
12. Zancolli EA, Goldner LJ, Swanson AB. Surgery of the spastic hand in cerebral palsy: report of the committee on spastic hand evaluation. J Hand Surg Am 1983;8(5 Pt 2):766–72.

13. Wolf TM, Clinkscales CM, Hamlin C. Flexor carpi ulnaris tendon transfers in cerebral palsy. J Hand Surg Br 1998;23(3):340–3.

14. Patterson JMM, Wang AA, Hutchinson DT. Late deformities following the transfer of the flexor carpi ulnaris to the extensor carpi radialis brevis in children with cerebral palsy. J Hand Surg Am 2010;35(11):1774–8.

15. Beach WRMD, Strecker WBMD, Coe JMD, et al. Use of the Green transfer in treatment of patients with spastic cerebral palsy: 17-year experience. J Pediatr Orthop 1991;11(6):731–6.

16. Thometz JGMD, Tachdjian MMD. Long-term follow-up of the flexor carpi ulnaris transfer in spastic hemiplegic children. J Pediatr Orthop 1988;8(4):407–12.

17. Van Heest AE, House JH, Cariello C. Upper extremity surgical treatment of cerebral palsy. J Hand Surg Am 1999;24(2):323–30.

18. Van Heest AE, Murthy NS, Sathy MR, et al. The supination effect of tendon transfer of the flexor carpi ulnaris to the extensor carpi radialis brevis or longus: a cadaveric study. J Hand Surg Am 1999;24(5):1091–6.

19. Hoffer MM, Perry J, Melkonian GJ. Dynamic electromyography and decision-making for surgery in the upper extremity of patients with cerebral palsy. J Hand Surg Am 1979;4(5):424–31.

20. Van Heest A, Stout J, Wervey R, et al. Follow-up motion laboratory analysis for patients with spastic hemiplegia due to cerebral palsy: analysis of the flexor carpi ulnaris firing pattern before and after tendon transfer surgery. J Hand Surg Am 2010;35(2):284–90.

21. Koman LA, Sarlikiotis T, Smith BP. Surgery of the upper extremity in cerebral palsy. Orthop Clin North Am 2010;41(4):519–29.

22. Tonkin MA. Thumb deformity in the spastic hand: classification and surgical techniques. Tech Hand Up Extrem Surg 2003;7(1):18–25.

23. Tonkin MA, Hatrick NC, Eckersley JRT, et al. Surgery for cerebral palsy part 3: classification and operative procedures for thumb deformity. J Hand Surg Br 2001;26(5):465–70.

24. House JH, Gwathmey FW, Fidler MO. A dynamic approach to the thumb-in palm deformity in cerebral palsy. J Bone Joint Surg Am 1981;63(2):216–25.

25. Van Heest AE. Surgical technique for thumb-in-palm deformity in cerebral palsy. J Hand Surg Am 2011;36(9):1526–31.

26. Smeulders M, Coester A, Kreulen M. Surgical treatment for the thumb-in-palm deformity in patients with cerebral palsy. Cochrane Database Syst Rev 2005;(4):CD004093.

27. Rayan GM, Saccone PG. Treatment of spastic thumb-in-palm deformity: a modified extensor pollicis longus tendon rerouting. J Hand Surg Am 1996;21(5):834–9.

28. Wenner SM, Johnson KA. Transfer of the flexor carpi ulnaris to the radial wrist extensors in cerebral palsy. J Hand Surg Am 1988;13(2):231–3.

29. Goldfarb CA, Calhoun VD. Hand and upper extremity therapy: congenital, pediatric & adolescent patients. Saint Louis protocols. 2nd edition.

30. James MA, Bagley A, Vogler JBIB, et al. Correlation between standard upper extremity impairment measures and activity-based function testing in upper extremity cerebral palsy. J Pediatr Orthop 2015. [Epub ahead of print].

31. Hoffer MM, Perry J, Garcia M, et al. Adduction contracture of the thumb in cerebral palsy. a preoperative electromyographic study. J Bone Joint Surg Am 1983;65(6):755–9.

32. Davids JR, Sabesan VJ, Ortmann F, et al. Surgical management of thumb deformity in children with hemiplegic-type cerebral palsy. J Pediatr Orthop 2009;29(5):504–10.

# Index

*Note:* Page numbers of article titles are in **boldface** type.

Hand Clin 32 (2016) 431–433
http://dx.doi.org/10.1016/S0749-0712(16)30051-8
0749-0712/16/$ – see front matter

# *Moving?*

## *Make sure your subscription moves with you!*

To notify us of your new address, find your **Clinics Account Number** (located on your mailing label above your name), and contact customer service at:

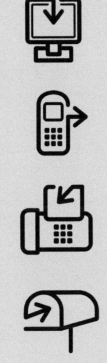

**Email: journalscustomerservice-usa@elsevier.com**

**800-654-2452** (subscribers in the U.S. & Canada)
**314-447-8871** (subscribers outside of the U.S. & Canada)

**Fax number: 314-447-8029**

**Elsevier Health Sciences Division**
**Subscription Customer Service**
**3251 Riverport Lane**
**Maryland Heights, MO 63043**

*To ensure uninterrupted delivery of your subscription, please notify us at least 4 weeks in advance of move.

Printed and bound by CPI Group (UK) Ltd, Croydon, CR0 4YY

03/10/2024

01040382-0011